Mindful Healing

DR AFROSA AHMED

The founder of **MindfulDoc**

Mindful Healing

5 Simple Steps to Transform Your Life

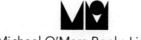

Michael O'Mara Books Limited

First published in Great Britain in 2024 by
Michael O'Mara Books Limited
9 Lion Yard
Tremadoc Road
London SW4 7NQ

A CIP catalogue record for this book is available from the British Library.

This product is made of material from well-managed, FSC®-certified forests and
other controlled sources. The manufacturing processes conform to the environmental regulations of the country of origin.

ISBN: 978-1-78929-662-4 in hardback print format
ISBN: 978-1-78929-692-1 in trade paperback format
ISBN: 978-1-78929-664-8 in ebook format

1 2 3 4 5 6 7 8 9 10

This book contains advice including instructions that are *FOR GUIDANCE ONLY*
and should not be relied upon as an alternative to professional advice from either
your doctor or a registered specialist. You are strongly recommended to consult a
doctor if you have any medical or other physical concerns. Neither the publisher
nor the author can accept any responsibility for any consequences that may follow
if such specialist advice is not sought.

Cover design by Natasha Le Coultre
Designed and typeset by Claire Cater
Printed and bound by CPI Group (UK) Ltd, Croydon, CR0 4YY

www.mombooks.com

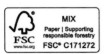

MIX
Paper | Supporting
responsible forestry
FSC® C171272

Dedication

To all my patients: thank you for trusting me with your life stories. The art of medicine starts and ends with you.

To all my students, whose energy and pursuit for knowledge kept me youthful and invigorated.

To my friends and relatives, nearest and dearest: you kept me sane and motivated.

To the pillar of the past, my parents and brother, whose sacrifice and support led me to where I am today.

To the gift of my present, my dear husband, whose friendship and love have given me the world and its entirety.

And to the promise of the future, my boys, and to all future generations, for whom this book was really written. Through this book, I hope to remain close to you.

Lastly, eternal gratitude to the Architect and Creator of the Universe.

Contents

Introduction

'As long as you are breathing there is more right with you than wrong with you, no matter what is wrong.'

Jon Kabat-Zinn

What's the point? No really, what's the point of all this? Of the things we do. What gets you up in the morning? Let's face it, we've all had these thoughts at one time or another. Nothing like hitting that snooze button in the morning and questioning your existence at the thought of repeating yesterday's activities. The answer? Hope.

There is some sort of motivation to get us out of bed after mind-numbing scrolling on our phones the night before. After hundreds of consultations as a doctor, seeing patients from all walks of life with their problems, I understand the business of people. You want to engage in something to change your emotional state. That's the point of it all. You're hopeful that by doing certain things you can change how you feel. For example, going to work will give you money, so you can buy tangible things to look good and then feel good or things that help you survive, like food and shelter. Getting up to get the kids to school fulfils a sense of duty and accomplishment and gives you time to do something else. Once that feeling has passed, you're looking for the next *thing* to experience happiness and joy – which for the most part is lacking, or appears to be lacking. The reality is that life is about engaging in a series of activities to change how you're feeling inside.

For some, there may be another purpose – religion, spirituality, humanitarianism and so on – but the basic principle is the same. Your motivation in life is to feel good and/or avoid suffering and pain. But is it possible to feel good now? Do you always have to wait till Monday to start afresh? Absolutely not. That is the limit you have placed on yourself, in your own mind, with your own inner voice.

So how does this programme work? As with all my patients, we first need to gain a thorough understanding of where you are at. You need to undergo a 360-degree life analysis that centres on your thoughts, because these are ultimately what drives your actions. Too often, people focus on changing the action first, assuming that that will change their thoughts. But in any wellbeing programme changing the thoughts must come first. For example, you want to lose weight and you decide to go on a diet, cutting out certain food groups or restricting the number of calories or perhaps exercising more. This can last for only a limited number of days or weeks – months at best. This is why diets do not work. If they did, the diet industry would not be so profitable. Without understanding what causes you to overeat, your thoughts around food, your relationship with food, how you use food to make you feel better, weightloss programmes will never be successful. The 'diet' part of it is the last step, not the first.

This is the purpose of the first part of the book: getting to know you. When I want my patients to engage in a programme that results in treatment or prevention of a disease or illness, that programme must be one that fits in with their lifestyle. By this I mean one that is doable, that considers their responsibilities and roles, such as their employment, their family setup, their likes and dislikes. We call this holistic medicine. Patients are less likely to follow the guidance they are given when a programme is generalized rather than personalized and doesn't consider them as a unique individual. A wellbeing programme is not meant to be difficult; it should fit in naturally, without feeling like a strenuous effort. If you start hating this process, then something has gone fundamentally wrong.

My interest is in healing. Throughout my journey as a medical doctor, I explored various methods in trying to help people feel better. To do this, I forced myself to step outside of the NHS – not because of criticisms of this wonderful institution, but because catering for the entire UK population understandably presents limitations in terms of time and resources. Unfortunately, modern-day medicine has limited focus on prevention. While there is a growing movement to incorporate prevention into healthcare, there remains a significant amount of work to do.

There was no specific life event that set me on a path to explore ways in which people can heal. I simply set about this journey to help my patients. I felt frustrated that I could not give them more; I wanted to understand their stories in more depth, and to get to know them on a personal level. This was just not possible within the confines of NHS consultations. The treatments we were offering as doctors did not go far enough and did not fully utilize the mind–body approach.

I looked into a variety of other wellbeing programmes, from CBT to hypnosis, emotional freedom technique (EFT) to acupuncture. But it was really mindfulness that resonated most strongly with me. And so, it is mindfulness that I use in this book's programme, which is discussed in the middle chapters. To ensure that you stick with the programme, and that it connects not only to your heart and your soul but also to your mind, I draw on scientific evidence to convince you of its benefits.

The final section of the book aims to ensure that the programme's journey does not come to an end but instead represents more of a beginning, to the rest of your life. We're not interested in short-term changes, but rather in lifelong changes. You need a programme that allows you to weather all the storms in your life, not one that offers a temporary fix. Here, I share with you the five steps, or building blocks, to help you achieve this. These five steps – also known as CAMPS: Character; Anchor in Awareness; Mastering the Mind; Pathway to Healing; Science of Stress and Self-Care – are at the heart of this unique wellbeing programme.

As a doctor, as an educator, as a mentor and as a fellow human who has seen an alarming increase in mental-health problems and wants to bring about lasting change, I'm so excited and honoured to be sharing this journey with you.

Dr Afrosa Ahmed

How to Use this Book

One thing I have learned from thousands of interactions with my patients is that any advice given needs to be simple and must fit in with the patient's beliefs for them to incorporate into their lives. It is unrealistic to just tell people to change their lifestyle and expect them to get on with it. There must be an educational element to the advice given, explaining the risks and benefits and exploring any ideas and concerns the patient may have.

So, for this guide I have adopted a prescriptive approach but one that details the theory and principles of mindfulness, backed by scientific evidence. I hope you will fully embrace these principles. There is no 'one size fits all' approach. At various points throughout this programme, you will need to reflect on the barriers in your life that are stopping you from implementing the practice described; you'll need to try different approaches, adjust and readjust where necessary.

In his 1960 book *Psycho-Cybernetics*, plastic surgeon Maxwell

Maltz noticed that it would take about twenty-one days for a patient to get used to their new image following surgery. Similarly, patients who had a limb amputated would feel that their limb was still there for twenty-one days before they got used to the fact that they no longer had an arm or leg. Building on this, Maltz observed himself that it took a minimum of twenty-one days to form a new habit. His work is now widely propagated, but it's important to note that word 'minimum': while everybody loves numbers – and numbers can make us feel we can achieve a goal – Dr Maltz said that twenty-one days is just the minimum time required.

Expectation is extremely important in any wellbeing programme. Attaching targets or numbers to the attainment of goals will inevitably lead to disappointment because the reality is that 'stuff' happens in our lives. You may set out to get things done but sometimes events beyond your control mean these things must be put off for a while. That's life.

During counselling for weightloss, the first question people usually ask is how long it will take until they see results. This is a normal thought process for someone who lives most of their life in a goal-setting mode. But here on this programme the goal is to fully embrace the principles of mindfulness, of which patience is a fundamental pillar that I will discuss further later in the book. I cannot tell you that in X number of weeks you'll notice a change. No doubt changes will occur if you follow the programme, but you must let them happen in their own time. The key is to notice that they're happening. Naturally, your mind will not always be comfortable with this, because for as long as it can remember it has been driven by goals and targets. This will not be the only time it feels uncomfortable. This whole programme will challenge your beliefs.

As doctors, we practise evidence-based medicine, which

means that we apply the best research to the care we provide our patients. This guide is based on the well-respected and renowned scientific work of Jon Kabat-Zinn and Dr Mark Williams. I would also acknowledge the Mindfulness Now programme, which is certified by the British Psychological Society. I have modified it, however, to make it more patient-friendly while keeping the core values.

The format of the guide is that every week there is some theory to read, because you are much more likely to be emotionally invested and motivated to do the work if you understand the concepts behind it. In addition, there will be some reflective work to do, like journalling. The final work to do each week is a daily meditation. I strongly encourage you to also review the previous weeks.

The principles of mindfulness include patience, compassion and loving-kindness. This is just a guide so allow flexibility in the plan. While goal-setting allows you to progress, be aware that it can also mean you neglect to notice the small changes, which are hugely significant. Goals can become obsessive and goal-setting can paradoxically restrict your happiness, as your internal nervous system goes into overdrive and soon you're feeling overwhelmed.

Your Weekly Challenge

The guide is laid out over five weeks, and each week of the programme contains five chapters outlining the theory work and then the week's meditations. (You will see that five is a number I repeat often during this programme: there are five working days in the week, five theory chapters and five meditations; the word CAMPS is made of five letters ...) **Each week will include the following tasks:**

◇ Reading: embedding the theory to understand the why – twenty minutes daily.

◇ Formal meditations: putting the theory into practice – ten minutes daily.

◇ Informal meditations: super-boosters to charge your self-development and enforce lifelong habits.

But free yourself of the idea of expectation. If Week One takes three weeks instead of one week, then that is your reality. Your life is different and everyone is an individual. Be kind and compassionate to yourself if the programme takes longer; it's more than OK. It does not mean that you are a failure or that you are not good at it. The key is to persevere, as you may have more work to do than someone else. Your life may be a bit more complicated, or you may be at a stage in your life where lots of challenges are happening. Recognize this. Accept it. Work with it.

Breathe. Mindfulness is like a gym for the mind. The more you practise it, the stronger your mind will be – which will manifest in various aspects of your life. It is very much dose dependent: the more you put in, the more you will get out. The one goal I would allow you in the first week is to evaluate how you can incorporate this programme into your daily routine.

Tools Required for this Programme

◇ Mind

◇ Breath

◇ Commitment

◇ Willingness

We're in this for the long haul, not just for a temporary solution for a few days or weeks at best. As you go through this book, highlight, annotate in the margins and make notes. Remember: this is like an exam, but the exam is your life.

Doctor's Prescription:
Commitment

Do not berate yourself for having had limited success with other programmes you've tried previously. None of them was a waste of time or effort. Each of those steps led you here. You are exactly where you need to be. This is no coincidence. However, one thing I require as your mentor and guide on this journey is commitment.

Commitment means different things to different people. Whether you commit five minutes a day or forty minutes, each minute spent on this programme is a win because it is a minute spent emerging from yesterday's habits and building new ones. You will notice me repeat this phrase often throughout the programme: there is no right, there is no wrong. There is no minimum commitment, no maximum commitment – just constant commitment.

I would like you to list some things you can do to allow you to commit yourself to this programme. For example, waking up fifteen minutes earlier, putting a time limit on social media or TV, notifying the rest of the household not to disturb you for thirty minutes, or putting your phone and any other devices away for twenty minutes. Gradually, throughout the programme, you will build up your commitment not because your doctor told you to but because joy and a wonderful array of other benefits begin to ripple in your life. You will naturally just crave more.

Introducing the Five
Simple Steps: CAMPS

For me, the idea of camping evokes warm childhood memories of a time when life was so much more … uncomplicated. Camping involved physical activities, creating social bonds, conversations around a campfire, listening to one another and developing essential life skills. While erecting the camp, various obstacles forced you to think critically and work together with others, fostering a sense of appreciation and developing your own inner survival skills. Being surrounded by nature gave a sense of stillness, while the vast depths of the forest represented the unknown and a sense of adventure, and fear, of what lurked beyond – very much like the journey of life.

The camp provided shelter from the elements of the weather, as well as safety from the surroundings. I will always cherish that feeling of achievement at having erected a successful camp. I have used the powerful symbolism of camping as an accomplishment to form this self-healing guide.

Setting up a successful camp involves several steps. First, you must prepare the area to ensure that it is flat and free from danger, away from hazards, while foreseeing any risks such as flooding or dismantling. To assemble your tent effectively and ensure that it is stable, you need a manual. The person who has written the manual must be a qualified expert and their instructions should be clear and based on successful past attempts. The manual should include advice on how to provide your camp with extra stability in the case of extreme weather.

This analogy incorporates all the elements of how I have written my guide. I will help you prepare yourself to start building your own camp. I will guide you to erect your tent and, more importantly, to ensure that it stays with you – providing shelter from whatever life throws your way. If there are moments of extreme turbulence, this guide will show you how to manage them. The guide begins with preparing the ground and will finish with the tools for a lifelong journey of self-empowerment and healing. The power of the programme lies in commitment, awareness and repetition. It is for anyone who can think and can breathe.

WEEK ONE:

CHARACTER

The core theme of this book is simple. The wellbeing programme centres around the idea of CAMPS. We do this by making a clearing to establish the camp and then building it, ensuring it is tailored to you and strong enough that it will withstand challenges.

The purpose of Week One is to identify the obstacles in your life that are preventing you from establishing change. If these obstacles are present, you may still notice some changes when undertaking a wellbeing programme but they will be short-lived. So, let's start clearing and cleansing.

This programme starts with the most important discovery of all: you. Learn who you really are and then uncover the tools to become who you want to be.

Here are some skills that you will learn
to cultivate this week:

Self-awareness

**Activating your 'inner tools' to
overcome challenges and emotions**

Emotional intelligence

Goal-setting

Introducing ... You

How would I start a patient consultation? I would begin by asking an open question: 'How can I help you today?' Hopefully the patient would then start to tell their story. However, when you see a doctor, you often have limited time. And this is the beauty of this book. We are in no hurry here; we go at your pace. There are no limitations at this moment.

My second question for you is: 'Why are you here?' Perhaps you have a problem or problems that are sufficiently impacting on your life for you to go and buy this book? Most problems do not arise in an instant but are an accumulation of other problems, over time. If you were to come to me and talk about your headaches I would need to know about your lifestyle, your triggers, the things that make the headaches worse and those that make them better. I would want to gain a full story – your story.

Similarly, you must do some groundwork before you embark on a wellbeing programme. The first step of this programme is to answer some more fundamental questions. Who are you? This type of questioning can sound daunting, as there is no definite answer; and you might think it seems too much at this time of the day. But I'm not asking you to lie on the doctor's couch and vocalize your innermost feelings.

To answer questions about who you are, you need to create a space where you feel safe and not judged. This is a skill I've learned over time. After all, I am expecting people who have never met me to tell me their innermost thoughts and answer sensitive, personal questions. So, I need to create a space where they feel they can trust me, without me labelling them or berating them. This is the fundamental principle of a doctor–patient relationship: trust. For you to undertake this process now you must trust me and, more importantly, trust yourself, without fear of judgement … not from me, but from you.

There are eight million humans on this planet, each one with their own identity, likes and dislikes. However, throughout history, human needs have essentially been the same. Every human has a physical need to eat, drink and breathe, as well as a need for shelter and clothing for protection. They also share a love for social and emotional connection, a striving for happiness and fulfilment and a need to have meaning in life. These later qualities may not be achievable, for whatever reasons, whether it's a lack of financial or other resources such as education or more personal barriers to accessibility. These unmet needs can lead to a host of symptoms such as loneliness, anxiety and sadness; or, worse, the belief that the needs are not important and can be substituted with something else.

So how does someone get to know their self? You are made up of years of experiences and interactions; your beliefs and your values have changed over time. But your needs remain constant, just as they did for your ancestors over the centuries. There has been no exam or college class to help you know yourself, detailing how you react to certain situations or to certain people. No school does this work. There are adult courses, but only if one seeks them. Yet ideally the actual work should take place in our formative, adolescent years, at school, in the context of a compulsory mind–body wellbeing programme – much like learning the alphabet.

So, one useful tool to answer the question of who you are is to undertake a life inventory. You could do this by journalling. However, if you are new to this journey even journalling may be quite difficult to begin with. I like to teach my patients and students with prompts. I did this with my first-year students at UCL Medical School in London. They were fresh-faced, just out of sixth form, and the group that I taught was called Clinical and Professional Practice (CPP). In their very first session, instead of the usual team-building activity, I undertook a group meditation, much to their surprise. But to their credit, they gave it a go. That was all I wanted – for them to start exploring meditation and experience it. I did not expect them to start meditating daily. However, the hope was that in later years when they were feeling stressed as medical students or junior doctors they would remember what I had taught them, and that it would provide a way for them to cope in a very demanding and stressful field.

I taught my CPP group that up until now they had worked competitively against each other to get to where they are. But what I wanted for them now was to start working together, being mindful of one another; to view their peers as supporters rather than as competitors. Despite all the negative press about the plight of doctors in the NHS, it is through teaching that you feel hope. I have never underestimated the impact that teaching – and in particular having inspiring teachers – can have on others. I think it is a profession that can make a lasting impact on a person's life. Much like being an author can.

Let me guide you through this first process. A life inventory encompasses self-reflection and analysis. This is not something frightening and, as with anything in mindfulness, there is no right or wrong way to do it. It does not require you to make meaning of anything but rather to discover what's important to you. Think of the ways that you have adopted so far that have helped you, as well as processes that have not worked in the past and so can be left behind.

Essentially, you are studying your life history. Why is history important? To understand what led to the current moment, you need to understand what led you here. This is the same approach that you need to move forward in your life, to avoid making the same mistakes and to understand what factors might lead you to repeat those mistakes.

Doctor's Prescription:
Making a Mindful Life Inventory (Life Journal)

Set aside some uninterrupted time to reflect on some key areas:

1) Identify what is most important to you. For example, family, career, health, weight, relationships.

2) Outline your achievements so far – personal, professional, emotional and so on. For example, improving your resilience or patience.

3) Note any major events in your life at present or in the future. A house move, project deadline, or family visit, for instance.

4) Make a list of all the activities and responsibilities you have in a typical week. This might include cooking, golf, eating out, work ... You could do this as a diary with hourly time intervals and fill it in over the course of one week.

For each of the above, highlight in three different colours:

1) The things you enjoy, that bring you happiness.

2) The things that make you feel anxious, stressed or tired.

3) Any of those that are beyond your control – for example, losing a job because the company has collapsed.

The purpose of this activity is to approach your life in a mindful way. By not paying attention to those activities that are beyond your control, you can release the energy you invest in them and instead immerse yourself more in activities that elevate your mood. Find ways to devote more time to them.

Try to find a different way to approach those activities that have a negative impact, or outsource them if you have the ability. If this is not possible, use the principles of mindfulness outlined later in this book. Notice the negative feelings you have and try to counteract them with some deep breathing or a short mindfulness practice. You could mentally reframe the event. If it is seeing someone who has caused you pain in the past, reframe it as: 'This will be over soon. Whatever they say, I will not dwell on it but go about my day noticing all the positive things in my life. I will not let one person have control over how I feel.'

The overarching lesson here is to begin to develop your own compass regarding your life triggers and pleasures, and in time learn to use the tools within you to overcome them. Every month or so, re-evaluate this list. Your life will begin to change. In time, you will notice that the joy-bringing activities you have highlighted will be greater in number and there will be fewer of those activities associated with negative feelings.

Edit this inventory often. Over a three-month period, you will appreciate the changes in your life. Look at your list at the end of the first month, the end of the third month and at the end of six and twelve months. The significant changes you will see will really motivate you to stay with the programme, as a lifelong commitment.

Principles of Mindfulness

Mindfulness has gained a lot of attention, especially in the Western world, but there are pros and cons to this. People now associate it with a ten-minute app or simple breathing exercises. When a concept becomes mainstream there is a risk of it becoming diluted. While this new popularity is great for awareness, the essence of mindfulness becomes lost. To gain the most from this phenomenon, you need to learn about the theory and core principles. Mindfulness is a relatively simple practice but it is rooted in centuries of wisdom and teaching.

Jon Kabat-Zinn, a professor of medicine who developed the renowned mindfulness-based stress reduction (MBSR) programme during the 1980s, set the groundwork for modern-day mindfulness being integrated into Western medicine and psychology. He talks about the principles of mindfulness, which have become universal. Building on this, I like to think of the pillars of mindfulness as the following:

1. Being
2. Patience
3. Observation
4. Non-judgement
5. Acceptance
6. Non-attachment
7. The novice

Let's take each one in turn.

Being

This is essentially mindfulness. To be present in the 'now' moment. Rather than getting caught up in the negative past or preoccupied with the uncertain future, you deal with reality. The only real moment is the present moment. So much of your time can be spent on yesterday or tomorrow that you miss out on the opportunities of today. Being present allows you to heighten your senses, so you gain understanding of how you respond to situations and are therefore able to manage them more effectively. Rather than just surviving and getting through the day, you adopt a mindset of enjoying each moment as it presents. You no longer live your life in fear.

Patience

Our default mode has become the 'doing' mode: striving for things, and wanting things to happen now or imminently. As you become increasingly addicted to apps such as TikTok or YouTube shorts and Instagram reels, your patience automatically decreases as you grow used to short, quick bursts of information that give you a quick dopamine fix.

However, you must remind yourself that making significant changes in your life takes time, and that there are processes that are beyond your control. As a result, there will be moments when you will just have to let things unfold. This is similar to the adage about a watched pot not boiling any faster. You need to let the process happen and trust that the outcome will be beneficial.

Mastering patience takes time, as the world you live in constantly sends the message that everything should be quick and instantaneous. However, being impatient will cause the mind to be agitated and lead to feelings of frustration. Learn to stand back, let things be and cultivate patience.

Observation

Observing one's thoughts and feelings is the central tenet of mindfulness. Awareness itself is enough to overcome negative feelings. However, observation needs to be from a safe place without judgement and self-criticism. Just observe your thoughts and feelings without getting caught up in them or taking a forceful approach and trying to change them.

You may wish to note down your observations of thoughts and feelings, especially if a stressful event is coming up. This process allows you to spot patterns. For example, if you know that every time you have an upcoming meeting you develop an acidic sensation in your upper abdomen, or a tense jaw or sweaty palms, you can incorporate a simple mindfulness practice so that those feelings do not escalate and overwhelm you. The idea is to be aware of your reaction and take control before the event.

This simple practice of observation and non-judgement allows you to develop resilience and the ability to handle events in a healthier way.

Non-Judgement

Non-judgement is a trait that is quite difficult to cultivate because you are so used to judging. Whether you judge yourself, other people, or situations, the need to label events or feelings has become automatic to most of us. To begin with, you will be in the habit of labelling even during meditation practice. For example, when you hear people talking on the road outside, your mind will automatically want to attach a story to that conversation. You might start to visualize the people, what they are wearing and what they look like. Soon you're caught up in irrelevant thoughts.

Non-judgement fosters kindness and compassion; by releasing yourself of the need to form an opinion, you become much more open and aware of situations. For your own mental wellbeing, releasing judgement from yourself – which is often self-critical – will improve your self-esteem.

Acceptance

Many of these principles are intertwined with each other. Acceptance is a close companion of patience, non-judgement and observation. Acceptance does not mean that you become apathetic or resigned to whatever life throws your way. It means acknowledging where you are in life, your thoughts, your feelings, without fear. In this safe space of open acceptance, you cultivate an improved relationship with yourself. Rather than trying to suppress your feelings or ignore them, adopting an accepting attitude will allow you to deal with them better.

Non-Attachment

You are constantly bombarded with the message that tangible objects will make you happy – whether it's a new holiday, a new item of clothing, or a new house. Well, no doubt those things can give us joy, but it is temporary. Attaching yourself to them to find happiness means you will never experience true, holistic wellbeing. While such things are also an essential part of life, there is a danger of obsessively wanting more. For instance, you might enjoy your new phone for a while until the next model comes out. The pursuit of happiness in this way is superficial and creates stress and anxiety as you think that without these things you will not experience joy. If this were true, then no millionaire in the world would have any mental-health problems and no person living in poverty would ever experience moments of joy.

Non-attachment also means to release yourself of goals and expectations. There are times when you need to set yourself targets – at work, for example. However, you do not need to adopt this approach in every aspect of your life. In meditation, you free yourself from any expectations and just accept what is in that moment. By releasing yourself from any targets you will automatically notice how relaxed you feel.

Try this with your family: rather than having to be somewhere at a set time, with everyone expected to wear certain clothes and with activities scheduled, have one event where you literally go with the flow. You will notice how freeing yourself and others of those boundaries means you are not shouting at people or getting frustrated because your expectations are unmet. This open space will foster a calmness and clarity that will feel liberating.

Non-attachment means finding a deeper sense of inner peace, rather than your happiness being attached to people or outcomes or objects. It also allows you to start to feel happiness now without waiting for X event to happen.

The Novice

This is perhaps my most favourite principle of all and is also referred to as the beginner's mind. It means approaching situations with a fresh curiosity, leaving any preconceptions or baggage behind. This is why children can learn things such as a new language at a fast pace – because they are a blank slate. They soak up knowledge like a sponge without discrimination or resistance. Leave behind whatever ideas you have heard about mindfulness and approach this course as a novice.

Doctor's Prescription:
Reminders

Mindfulness is the tool you will use to enforce changes in your life and ensure they are lasting. This is a chapter worth spending time on. Here are some practical strategies:

○ Make a note of the seven mindfulness principles – on your phone or somewhere you see daily, like a bathroom mirror. Familiarity is key.

o Identify the principles you need to work on the most and choose one to focus on. For example, Being.

o Think of ways you can strengthen this principle in your life. For example, 'I am going to check in with myself every hour and notice where my attention is. If I am overthinking, I will use mindful breathing to ground myself.'

o Supplement your knowledge of mindfulness with extra reading or podcasts. This could be related to the whole principle of mindfulness, or just one aspect of it. Adjust this strategy to your learning style – you could watch a short TED Talk on a Tube ride, or listen to a podcast in the car or while cooking, or do some bedtime reading.

o Remind yourself this is a lifelong skill and as such is a process that stays with you, not a practice you do for a short while before moving on.

Beware of the Traps

A mindful way of life means living in the present moment in a non-judgemental way. Sounds simple. However, living in the present moment has now become an alien concept to many of us and something that seems difficult to do. In fact, you may live in every moment *but the now*.

As well as letting go, become aware of the traps of the mind that will consume you. Liberating yourself from these will take time but is essential to personal growth. Every now and then, you will find these traps waiting for you, begging you to come back. Through mindful meditation, your desire to be controlled by these will just simply fall away.

The Time Trap

The reality is that you spend a lot of your time on past events. Events such as conversations that happened earlier in the day, and interactions with your colleagues or family, often replay on repeat. Especially at night, or when you have a quiet moment to yourself, you get caught up with thoughts of the past. Your mind loves to remember even the tiniest of details. When you give these details attention, they become bigger than they were.

The other way that you spend your life is thinking about the future. Energy goes into planning and analysing events and then trying to predict their outcome. You get so caught up in trying to pre-empt every single possible scenario, and often go back to re-strategizing the plans. This approach makes you feel overwhelmed and you end up suffering from decision fatigue. Essentially what you are doing is trying to protect yourself – and that is the job of the mind. Your mind is less concerned with joy and happiness and more with survival.

The cumulative effect of spending your time in the past or the future is that you become devoid of contentment; your mind is unable to switch off, unable to relax, and your emotional and physical needs will not be met. Instead, burnout, fatigue, stress, overthinking and anxiety become the default mode. You live in a state of stress rather than one of relaxation. This constantly heightened state of being can then manifest into physical illness and disease.

With mindfulness, you become aware of your thoughts in the present moment. Rather than burning energy thinking about the past and the future, being concerned with the present moment becomes the stabilizing force in your life. You have no control over the past; you cannot change it. You can try to manipulate the future, but the reality is that your predictions may not come true and that too is out of your hands. So, focus on what is certain. What is certain is the now moment, the present moment.

The Thinking Trap

You need a wellbeing programme that encompasses everything. Such a programme is possible, but only by addressing the way you think. Everything comes from your perception. Your ability to deal with events largely depends on how you view them. You have a choice. You can view them as negative and dwell on them, or you can see the good in these events. This could be difficult at first, especially if you are programmed to think in a certain way. However, viewing events in a positive light allows you to develop better coping mechanisms, which improves their outcome. Positive thinking improves resilience and allows you to have greater confidence, which enhances your self-esteem.

There is plenty of medical evidence that individuals who have a positive mindset experience a range of benefits, including reduced incidence of depression, lower blood pressure, a balance of blood-sugar levels, reduced risk of heart disease, a positive effect on weight and ultimately a longer life.

Once you become aware of your thoughts, you can catch yourself thinking negatively. You can break free from living your life and reacting to events as you have done in the past. Awareness is so powerful. In many instances just being aware of our thoughts and feelings is enough to enforce a change.

In some cases, however, you need to take an extra step. And that is that once you are aware of your thoughts you separate from them by creating space between you and the thought. By creating some distance, you gain a clearer perspective. The feeling of being overwhelmed, having scattered thoughts and losing oneself dissipates quite quickly with the practice of mindfulness.

You cannot change what you do not know. It's a well-known saying that insanity is doing the same thing but expecting different results. You need to understand what has led you to this moment. *I need to understand what has led you to this book.*

Thought → Action

Thought → Mindfulness →
Different action → Different outcome

Your thoughts shape your reality. They form the basis of your beliefs and in turn shape your actions. This is the 'why' of why you do things. Thoughts can be shaped by experiences, by cultures, by your own set of values. They can also be influenced by other people or things in your environment. Whatever the case, the reality is that you and no one else are in control of your thoughts. The thoughts belong to you. This is the heart of the programme. You change the way you think and perceive to bring about lasting change in your life.

So, decide here and now, in this moment. Will you continue to let external factors shape your thoughts? Or are you going to seize control? If you commit yourself to fostering positive thoughts, be aware of the negative ones that lead to fear and worthlessness.

Inner thoughts → Outer world

Putting space between your thoughts and observing them from a distance frees you from the grip your mind has over you. Free yourself also from the addiction of labelling thoughts. These thoughts are perceived as truth, but often you have added your own version of the truth and the outcome has become murky. In your mind you are the centre of the universe. If you shift to being *part of the universe, you will release the behaviours and thoughts that have resulted in toxic behaviour.*

The Doing Trap

To be still in body and in mind was a natural state of being when you entered this world but has now become an unnatural state. The internal chatter of our minds keeps us busy even when we may be physically resting. Have you ever taken a holiday but come back feeling like you needed another break? This is because your thoughts and mind did not take a holiday; they remained with your problems back home.

The preoccupied mind is not in a state of calm. The conscious act of being is no longer our default mode. The mind is like a rollercoaster, catching thoughts like a runaway train, inventing stories, adding interpretations to events. Soon you become totally engrossed in that story. This behaviour is addictive, like a thrill-seeking adrenaline rush. The need to label every thought with judgement becomes overwhelming, activating your sympathetic nervous system (see page 212).

The opposite of this doing mode is the being mode, which is an essential part of mindfulness. Rather than constantly being in a state where you are living your life by goals and targets, the being mode means simply staying in the present moment. It requires you to observe without reaction at that moment and without planning or predicting the future, which will overwhelm you, or revisiting the past and feeling deflated. The being mode is about acceptance and awareness, staying present and thereby reducing anxiety and stress and promoting wellbeing.

Freeing yourself from the mind and just being in a state of acceptance will lead to a state of peace and calm. Freeing yourself from the rollercoaster of thoughts frees you from expectations and the negative stories you have developed. Life is not complicated when you free yourself from the thoughts that have caused mental suffering. You enter a true state of freedom, which allows joy and a feeling of completeness.

Living in the present moment requires awareness. This is a harmony that can be achieved. Without being obsessed with time, you can breathe. Possibilities open up from a place of non-judgement, without the boundaries you have placed upon yourself.

To develop that stillness and freedom of thought, you utilize the power of meditation. Quietening the mind and just observing with presence will allow you to start to heal. Experiencing calmness, rather than your former state of needing to be doing something, will soon become addictive. In this new consciousness, infinite space becomes a space of growth. In time, this will break habits that have come to define you – the need to control, to overthink, to undermine yourself, to berate yourself.

Being mindful is about acceptance over resistance. Being and acceptance, however, do not mean surrendering as if you are a victim to the universe. Rather, they mean clarity and freedom to make wiser choices. There is certainly a time for doing in life, but you need to balance it with greater moments of being.

Doctor's Prescription:
Bring Awareness

The human brain has about 70,000 thoughts a day. Try to 'catch' some of them. Set an alarm every hour and note down what you are thinking. Then, see if there is a pattern. Are there more negative or positive thoughts?

What is your default mode of thinking? Remember that
these thoughts are not real and you do not have to let
them define you.

I am useless

I knew this
would end badly

I can't get motivated

Nothing goes
right for me

I am so tired of this

I can't do
anything right

I just want to
hide away

It's too much

I didn't need to
worry about it

I am dreading this
event but I am going to
look for the positives,
no matter how small

Actually, I am good at …

In my head it was
much worse

I am thinking about
all the times things
did work out

Conscious Coupling

Mindfulness has two parts. The formal part (also known as mindfulness meditation) and the informal part (for example, mindful walking, or mindful eating). While both parts are crucial, the actual repeated practice of informal mindfulness is what strengthens the outcome. Let's first focus on formal mindfulness meditation. The practice is amazingly simple. There are only two tools that are needed:

The breath + The mind

This means that any person who is alive and possesses the capacity to think can meditate. Therefore, this includes children, the immobile and those with chronic illnesses. You do not need a fancy studio, expensive props or special clothing. Meditation is the cheapest and most accessible form of therapy.

As a beginner, you may wish to follow a guided script. As

you become more experienced, you will become attuned to your feelings and use this insight to guide your meditation practice for that day. The most important factor to remember is that you free yourself from labels such as 'right' or 'wrong'. There is no one way to meditate. Here is a space for freedom; acknowledge the flow you are feeling in the moment and then go with it. You do not need to interpret any outcome, thoughts or feelings during the process. You do not need to try to make sense of anything. In this regard, meditation is an extremely safe and non-threatening practice.

Meditation requires only that you show up. As with anything new, your mind will try to resist; usually this resistance will be in the form of thoughts. Remember: if you want to free yourself from thoughts, then the solution is simply awareness. You are trying to prevent the mind from doing what it has been doing for years and years, which is what it believes is keeping you safe: repeating negative thoughts and being in every moment but the present.

Therefore, you need to be aware of when thoughts enter your mind during the practice. These can be thoughts such as:

- 'This isn't working.'
- 'I feel stupid.'
- 'Oh, I've got a pain now ...'
- 'I've got a lot to be getting on with.'
- 'I don't have time for this.'
- 'I've tried so many things; why is this going to be any different?'
- 'Nothing ever goes right for me; this isn't going to work either.'

This is the mind doing what it does best, keeping busy and stimulating those feelings of doubt and worthlessness. You are not your thoughts. When the mind uses these tactics, all you need to do is notice them and thank the mind for bringing them to your attention, rather than criticizing yourself and thinking that you are a failure.

As quickly as they enter your mind, the thoughts will leave. Just release them as if they were dandelions in the wind. The thoughts are light and have no effect on you; they just bounce off. At the beginning of a meditation routine, you may have these thoughts every thirty seconds – perhaps even more. Just continue to be aware of them. In time, they will become less frequent as you are able to master your thoughts, without getting caught up in them and allowing them to divert your attention.

Clothing

While you do not need to have any special clothing, I do advise you to wear something loose and comfortable, so the mind does not have a chance to use this as an excuse for grabbing your attention. While you want to remain relaxed, you do not want to fall asleep. This is very important. You need to retain attention and awareness throughout the practice. With that in mind, I would not advocate wearing anything associated with sleep, such as pyjamas, or doing this practice in your bed.

Surroundings

During a meditation, your senses will be heightened. Finding a quiet spot will help you to remain focused. Your mind loves to make connections. In this way, your bed is associated with sleeping and a study or computer room will be associated with working. This may also preoccupy your mind. While you are a novice, find a room where you will be calm and relaxed.

If you live with others, inform them that you need some time alone. Do not worry about what their perceptions or thoughts about you might be. To make sure you are not interrupted, turn off your mobile phone and any alerts such as a ring doorbell. To eliminate as much distraction as possible, it is advisable to close your eyes so you are not preoccupied with the world around you. Whether you do this along with music or not will be a personal preference, dependent on your own learning style. Some may find music a distraction, while others find it helps them to remain calm. I would avoid any music with words unless they form a guided meditation.

Posture

The best posture for you to retain your attention with the meditation is to sit upright, in a chair, with your feet flat on the floor, forming a connection with the ground. I like palms to face upwards as if in the receiving mode. Use cushions, blankets or whatever you need to make yourself comfortable. There is no right or wrong here; if you wish, you can lie on the floor, or in the garden. Find whatever works best for you.

Duration

The first step to any meditation is to focus on your breath. The duration of the practice is also flexible. Usually, I recommend starting slowly, with ten-minute sessions, working your way up to twenty minutes, forty minutes and then to an hour as a daily practice. Life is such that you can't plan every single aspect. Be it because of illnesses, work events, or holidays, there will be days you may be unable to meditate. That is fine. Acceptance is a huge part of the programme. Accept that, for today, this is how things will be.

Without judgement, the all-or-nothing concept is one of the most self-destructive concepts. The idea that you either put 100 per cent into something or it is deemed a failure is unrealistic. This idea arises because you have subscribed to the idea of perfection. But thinking that you will not gain anything if you don't meditate every day for one hour does not allow for life's uncertainties that come your way. It does not allow you to celebrate the small gains. Every achievement should be recognized. This approach will raise your vibration and your self-worth. Instead, if you have faced obstacles in establishing a meditation routine, re-evaluate why this has occurred. Rather than give up the idea of meditating, see what changes you can make tomorrow to help implement this practice.

Sometimes a simple mental shift is all that's required. For example, the way you brush your teeth, take a shower, find time to have breakfast, to exercise … You do these things because you recognize their importance. You find the time to do them. Viewing meditation as a life skill and essential for your own personal growth and development will help you to establish it as a regular practice. Once you understand its impact and how important it is, you will be able to find ways to readjust your schedule and fit it in. And schedules do not have to be so fixed. Your commitments on weekdays are different to your commitments at weekends. You may have additional roles at different times – for example, ferrying children around or visiting relatives. Factor these in. Maybe you need to meditate at a different time on the weekends, and for slightly less time. Make the effort to evaluate your life so that you can incorporate meditation regularly, no matter for how long.

It is also important to recognize that acceptance means that you do not place any expectations on meditation – that you must feel a certain way or expect a shift immediately after meditating. You have been living your life the same way for many years and it will take some time to now live your life differently. If changes occur – and they will in time – notice them and embrace them. Often the changes are small in the beginning but, as with anything, lots of small steps ultimately lead to large shifts in your life. Go into the meditation free of any fixed beliefs, but after the meditation observe any changes with an open mind and welcome them.

The Seven Basic Steps
of Meditation

1. Find a quiet spot to eliminate as much visual and auditory distraction.
2. Get comfortable in an upright posture, palms facing upwards.
3. Close your eyes and start to focus on your breath.
4. Be aware of thoughts as an observer, just watching them float by.
5. Continue to focus on your breath for a time.
6. To bring the meditation to a close, bring your awareness back to the room and open your eyes.
7. Stay here as long as you wish before you go about your day.

Doctor's Prescription:
The Mind–Body Connection

I would like to show you that your thoughts can cause physical reactions in your body. This is a simple practice that many mindfulness practitioners undertake. I love the simplicity of it, yet there is overwhelming evidence of how our thoughts can have an impact on our physical being.

You can stand or sit down, close your eyes and start to relax by taking some deep breaths.

○ Imagine you are in your kitchen standing at the kitchen worktop.

○ You notice the bowl of fruit on the worktop with fresh yellow lemons.

○ Pick up one of the lemons in your hand and notice the weight of it, then feel the texture of the lemon peel with your fingers. The waxy, rubbery feeling.

○ Now take that lemon and place it on a cutting board, cut the lemon in half.

○ You immediately notice the lemon juice spilling out onto the board and you get a quick aroma of the lemon.

○ Take one half of the lemon and hold it to your nose, taking a deep inhalation of that citrus smell. Breathe in deeply.

○ Now open your eyes. What have you noticed? Is your mouth filled with saliva?

This exercise demonstrates the power of visualization. Even though there was no lemon, your body thought there really was. And as a result, a physical response occurred where saliva was discharged from the salivary glands under the tongue, into your mouth, through the salivary ducts. This simple yet powerful practice shows that when you start to master your thoughts, you can then be the master of your physical and mental health. If you start to think from a positive mindset then you can improve your physical parameters, such as heart rate and blood pressure, and other aspects of your wellbeing. The mind and body are not separate but one entity.

Meditations

As you go through the book, you will find various meditations. Each set is designed to reinforce the theoretical concepts of the week in which it appears. Aim to do each meditation at least once a day. You may feel that you want to focus on one meditation more than another, depending on how you are feeling or the events in your life. This is perfectly acceptable. You can stay with one meditation for many days or practise a new one each day during the week and repeat particular ones at the weekend. Likewise, you don't need to do the meditations in a specific order; simply choose one that resonates with you.

Meditations for Week One are designed to introduce you to the practice and to familiarize you with your breath while you stay present and tame the mind. Remember, these are skills that do not develop overnight; but once you have a strong grounding, your self-development will flourish.

Warning

Meditation is generally a safe practice, but it can at times exacerbate certain mental-health conditions, such as anxiety or depression, and certain forms of epilepsy and asthma. If you have a pre-existing mental-health condition, please consult your doctor before you start the programme. Meditation is not a replacement for medical treatment but can be a powerful complement.

Before undergoing a formal mindfulness meditation practice, ensure that you are in a safe location that does not require your full attention, as at times you will be in a deep relaxation state. You should not meditate while operating machinery or driving.

Mindful Breathing (1)

You will begin this mindfulness meditation journey with that which brought you into this world: your breath. Learn to befriend it. You will begin to spend a lot of time with one another in a state of consciousness.

1. Find a comfortable seat and sit with your spine tall, your shoulders and neck relaxed, your palms on your lap, ideally facing upwards, and begin to close your eyes.
2. Start to notice your breath, breathing in and out for as long as each breath needs, not forcing the breath to be in any way but accepting it fully. This is the opening

of any state of relaxation: watching and noticing your breath and returning to it if your mind wanders.

3. As long as there is breath, continue this journey to notice, to see, to feel, to listen, to just be. You are the watcher, the observer and the witness; no other person can take this position of privilege.

4. Remain here and rest. With that awareness, there is a sense of freedom. This journey is the beginning but is limitless as you rest in this vast spaciousness of awareness.

5. While you are feeling relaxed and open, the breath continues to provide a deep sense of contentment. Be grateful for each breath as you notice your chest expanding and your abdomen releasing, sensing the whole body moving with the tide of each breath.

6. Know there is nowhere else you need to be and nothing else you need to do; you have everything in this moment. All you need is right here and right now in this open acceptance. Repeat out loud, 'I am content.'

Your Constant Companion: The Breath

You will continue to build your awareness of the breath here. This is a fundamental pillar of mindfulness. By appreciating its continued presence in your life, you will begin to master the art of meditation.

1. Adopt a position to start your meditation and lower your gaze. Sit comfortably in a quiet place, with your spine elevated in a dignified position.

2. Start to bring attention to your breath and be mindful of the movement and changes of the breath. With every exhale, you will start to feel grounded and at peace.

3. Remain centred and remember that the weather around you may change but with the focus on the breath, you accept everything as it is.

4. Welcome everything at this moment. From this base, you will grow even further. There is no doing at this moment. You have permitted yourself to simply be.

5. Stay with your breath. Notice whatever is on your mind, but understand that nothing needs to be done about it. In this moment, thinking is not required for your healing.

6. Give your mind permission to rest. You will begin to feel at ease and stay in the moment. There is a freedom in resting and a feeling of deep contentment. There is no need to try to change anything. Everything is as it should be.

7. This is your true state. With each breath in and each breath out your constant companions.

Clarity in an Instant

You spend much of the time clouded. In your emotions, in your thoughts. This state does not allow you to progress or be clear about the goals in your life. This meditation will help overcome overthinking and self-doubt.

1. What are you feeling right now? Any strong emotions? Notice what has caught your attention,

which may also manifest as a physical sensation of discomfort or pain.

2. Recognize and acknowledge these things in turn, exploring with kindness.

3. Start to breathe into those areas, releasing tension and thoughts into the air, rather than involving yourself in them and creating a story that you know will consume you eventually.

4. Use the breath to regain clarity in your thoughts and emotions and take back control. Become aware of the stillness in this moment.

5. Instead of your troubles taking the weight, release your body to gravity. Just sinking to where you're sitting or lying, noticing the points of contact between your body and the floor or the chair.

6. There may be several thoughts on your mind again. Notice each one as it arises and let it pass right through you without getting caught up in its detail.

7. You feel a lightness now as with each breath the strong emotions release just as easily as they entered.

8. If for a moment you do get caught up once more in the stories of your mind, come back to the present moment with the breath.

9. Notice each inhale and each exhale, again and again and again for as long as necessary.

Coming Back

Our natural state is a place of peace and tranquillity. But you may feel you have not experienced this state in your life as often as you would have liked. Let us come back to it.

1. Begin to close your eyes and return through a state of mindfulness.
2. Be mindful of your breath, the movement, the changes in the sensations in your body. Make a commitment to stay here.
3. With every inhale and every exhale, you will begin to feel anchored and rooted.
4. In this peaceful state that you have cultivated, remind yourself that you have helpers. Recall anyone who has helped you; imagine them as if they were right in front of you, here and now. It could be a family member, a colleague, a neighbour or even a stranger.
5. Feel their support as a warmth like a blanket surrounding you. Thank all the helpers in your life. Smile at them as they smile at you. Remember that you are fully supported with the gift of helpers from far and wide.
6. Now visualize a bright shining ball of light, vibrant and glowing. Feel that light descend from the sky above to the centre of your heart.
7. Whatever direction the weather pushes and pulls you in, you can return to the light in your centre. The light will remain locked here as you go about your day.
8. Through mindful gratitude, your natural state will want to return to this safe place you have cultivated.

Alleviate Resistance

You can read this script to yourself while you do the practice, or you can record it and listen to it with some headphones. Alternatively, you may like someone else to read this to you.

However, this should be someone who does not evoke strong feelings and whose presence you find supportive. You may wish for them to record it and you listen back to it. Find whatever works for you. Remind yourself that in meditation there is no right or wrong; your experience is just that – your experience.

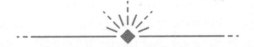

'Take a moment to settle your body as you intentionally take this time for yourself. I will guide you through a practice to relieve resistance. This could be resistance to something that you need to do, or blocks in your life that are preventing you from progressing, or a general feeling of being stuck.

In this practice, you are cultivating an alternative sense of openness and space. This could be a physical space or a space around difficult emotions. Let's begin.

Take a full breath in for two seconds; pause and then take a long breath out for five seconds. As you continue to breathe in, imagine breathing in positive energy that will revitalize your tired body. Take some deeper breaths in and ensure that each breath reaches every part of you, right down to the tips of each finger and the soles of both feet.

If your body wants to move or shift during the meditation, show it kindness and let it do so. There is no right or wrong in this moment.

Instead of the mind taking centre stage, as it usually does, let's focus on the other major organ that keeps you alive. The heart. This is situated on the left side of the chest. What feeling is there here?

You may be able to feel it beating now that you have placed your attention on it. Or there might be a fleeting sensation. Or there may be no feeling, as the heart carries on pumping blood around the body, minding its business, concerned only with the continuation of life. Your life.

As you continue to breathe in and breathe out, in gratitude, notice how you now feel a sense of ease from where you started. How resistance is beginning to melt away, now the heart has taken centre stage.

How are you feeling now? Check in fully. Are there still blocks? Areas you feel resistance, where the breath does not flow as naturally?

Mostly these blocks have been put there by you. Without dissecting how they got there or what they are, just notice their presence.

I would now like you to visualize these blocks as a wall in front of you. The size of the wall is completely up to you. If it seems large and insurmountable, then so be it. However, now that you are relaxed, with the power of visualization you will see that it is not as big as you imagined.

With each breath, you have gained strength. Notice the positive energy flowing through each artery and vein, in every single part of your body. You suddenly feel confident; there is nothing that you cannot overcome. Even the wall in front of you.

With each breath out, one brick in turn begins to fall away. Another brick falls effortlessly. A third, fourth, fifth ... Effortlessly, the wall is now half the size.

You already notice that the extent of your resistance reflects the size of the remaining wall. Suddenly you feel light. Your shoulders are loose, and your arms and limbs are relaxed. Even your mind begins to congratulate you.

Continue to take some more deep breaths as you tackle the remaining resistance. Now all that is left is a line of single bricks.

All that remains to do is to step over that line. That's it, just step over. And it is done. You look behind and you see the line of bricks. You thank the wall for the lessons that it has taught you, and tell it that you no longer need it.'

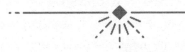

Informal Mindfulness Practice

Suggested time: ten minutes daily.

You have the theory to help you understand the work that is being done here and you have the mindfulness meditations. Those meditations are called formal mindfulness practices. They require you to set aside specific time to do them; they cannot be done in any old setting or at any old time.

Now meet the partner of formal mindfulness: the *in*formal mindfulness practice. This is the use of mindfulness in everyday activities. It involves giving your attention to thoughts and feelings in the present moment, wherever you are, whatever you are doing. So, informal mindfulness can be done while you are washing the dishes, walking, on a train, or talking to someone.

In a 2021 study focused on Australian medical students, behavioural research scientist Naomi Kakoschke and colleagues looked at informal mindfulness and its relation to wellbeing. Medical students are known to experience stress due to the demanding nature of their course. These students undertook a five-week mindfulness-based course and answered questions about how they felt before and after the course. The study found that the mental health of all participants improved, which also had a positive effect on their studies. The research concluded that there were particular improvements when students engaged in informal mindfulness practices compared to formal practices.

However, both are essential. Rather than letting your mind wander and getting lost in your story, stay present in whatever situation you are in. This will strengthen your formal mindfulness sessions, by building the foundation for awareness. Think of it as the warm-up, essential for the main match.

Mindful Breathing (2)

This week, the main star of your self-healing journey is the breath. Mindful breathing on its own is a powerful tool to bring you back to the present moment and ease stress, helping you feel relaxed. Try to befriend your breath and do this exercise daily. Start with ten minutes and build the time up gradually if you can.

1. Whatever you are doing, just pause – not physically but mentally. Notice your breath, wherever it happens to be – in your chest, your nose, your abdomen. Depending on what you are doing and where you are, if

your hands are free you may wish to put them on your chest or tummy to help you notice.

2. Observe your breath without judgement; you just want to get to know the breath. What is it doing? How does it feel? No need to change it; just pay attention.

3. As you do so for some time, your mind will take your attention off the breath. Let it. Then bring it back.

4. Pay attention to the cycle of breathing, in and out. The chest wall, up and down. The exchange of carbon dioxide out and nourishing oxygen in. Be thankful for the breath.

5. Stay in this moment for as long as you can.

End of Week One

By the end of this first week, through an in-depth understanding of your situation, you will have gained an appreciation of why, until now, your self-development has not progressed. Not just physically, but in terms of the thoughts you carry and hold, which you have used to make important decisions in your life. Now that you have dismantled, you are ready to build.

WEEK TWO:

ANCHOR IN AWARENESS

Before you can build your CAMPS, you need to ensure you have the essential tools the task requires. This week will focus on establishing such crucial components as compassion, gratitude and resilience.

Affection is key to any healing programme – and the most meaningful affection is the kind you give yourself. To build your camp, you must create a nurturing environment with kindness anchored in awareness.

Here are some skills that you will learn
to cultivate this week:

**Developing cohesive harmony
between your different
biological systems**

**Freeing yourself from the past to
move forward with your goals**

**Utilizing your body's natural
antidepressant pathway**

**Boosting your learning process to
ensure the theory is truly embedded**

The Beating Heart

Civilization has made huge advances thanks to the 'doing mode', in which the analytical mind is at the forefront. The doing mode is all about thinking and thoughts and it's in this mode that modern mankind spends most of its waking hours. In fact, when we want to make sense of something or prove anything to be true, the mind is always our first port of call. Things are much more likely to be accepted if they can be proved in a scientific or logical way.

We have a lot to thank the mind for. But with every yin, there is a yang – a connected and equal opposite. For the mind, it is the heart. Yet somewhere along the path of enlightenment taken by mankind, the heart has been forgotten.

The heart is a vital organ of every single human being. Your body is made up of different systems, such as the respiratory system, lymphatic system, the nervous system and musculoskeletal system. The heart is the centre of the circulatory system, whose function is to pump blood through the body to deliver oxygen and nutrients vital to your existence. All these systems operate every single second without any thought or input from yourself. They just are.

The Heart–Mind Connection

So far, we have discussed the mind–body connection, but in a 2001 scientific statement, the American Heart Association noted that a heart–mind connection exists. The autonomic nervous system, which is composed of the sympathetic and parasympathetic nervous systems, connects the heart and mind. The brain sends messages to the heart, but the heart is also able to send information back to the brain. It can do this through neurological processes but also via hormones, pressure waves and electromagnetically. For blood to travel quickly throughout your body to meet its needs, the body's circulatory system needs to be under pressure. Through its pumping action, and the expansion and contraction of blood vessels, the intricate system of the heart ensures that in one heartbeat much vital exchange can occur.

It is evident that the heart is a central part of your health and fitness, as exercise is often advocated for general wellbeing and for anyone with cardiovascular disease. It is well known that stress is also connected to the heart: chronic stress can lead to elevated heart rates and blood pressure, which can lead to illness. The heart is literally at the heart of your being.

When you feel strong emotions, such as a panic attack or anger, you will experience an elevated heart rate. Conversely, when you feel relaxed your heart rate decreases. This is a central principle of mindfulness. With the introduction of devices such as smart watches, you can easily keep track of these changes. When you are exercising or in a stressful situation, notice your heart rate and compare it to a situation where you are more relaxed, such as sitting down reading a book or just having a refreshing cup of herbal tea.

Heart-Based Living

Increasingly used in this modern-day era of holistic care is the term 'heart-based living', where you pay attention to your thoughts and feelings, through the heart, helping to make positive choices in your life. Rather than the mind controlling every aspect, heart-based living includes involving the heart as well as logic, in daily decisions. This does not cloud your judgement but rather brings qualities of compassion, patience and forgiveness that will reduce stress.

From our medical knowledge we know that stressors, when detected by the body's natural physiology, activate the fight and flight response, which increases blood pressure and heart rate, therefore directly affecting the heart. The 2004 INTERHEART study further elaborates on the link between heart disease and emotional stress. There is also growing evidence that those with positive psychological wellbeing have improved outcomes related to cardiovascular disease.

It could be said that the heart is more important than the brain – because when the brain dies, the heart will continue to beat; and in human embryology, the heart begins to beat even before the brain is developed. The heart also has its own magnetic field, which radiates outside the body and can be sensed by those around you. This is important, as many wellbeing programmes talk about the self. But you are not a lone entity in this world. Relationships and people are part of you. This can be a source of great stress or comfort. When we talk about wellbeing you must also appreciate the world around you.

Heart Coherence

Practising mindful techniques increases your heart's coherence, which then sends positive energy that can affect others. It is thought that the heart's energy can spread beyond your physical body by about a metre. The electromagnetic field of the heart is 5,000 times greater than the brain. Its impact is huge. Have you ever entered a room and immediately picked up on the energy?

Through increasing your heart's coherence, not only can you positively affect those around you but you are also less likely to be reactive to other people. By strengthening your emotional stability, you can ensure that people and events have less influence over you and that you can instead positively influence them.

To my dismay, wellbeing programmes often place insufficient focus on the heart. It is sadly neglected. Like its partner, the mind, the heart can be retrained, which can in turn affect your overall health. Increased awareness of the heart, in the same way that we pay attention to the mind, will alter the state of the whole body.

Doctor's Prescription:
Practising Heart Coherence

Greater heart awareness can happen just by focusing your attention to the heart, bringing it to the forefront of your mind. Make sure that your surroundings are the same you'd create for entering a meditative state. Try to sense an awareness of the heart beating and appreciation and gratitude for all that your heart does to keep you alive.

Increase the appreciation of your heart by placing your hands on it. This tactile stimulation is picked up by your nervous system, sending chemical messages to the brain to promote a feeling of calmness and relaxation.

Deep breathing will slow down the heart rate, which will aid your awareness of the heart 'brain'. Visualizing an event or person who brings you happiness will evoke a positive emotion in the heart; let a smile come across your face while you involve your entire being in this practice. Repeat this practice often so that you become reacquainted with your heart, even though it has been with you since birth.

Letting Go

Once you have identified your personal qualities and have taken the time to know what you like and dislike, without judgement, you can start to move on and freely let go. Presently in your life there are blocks, which can be physical or mental. It is these blocks that will prevent you from achieving any meaningful and lasting change. I have identified four blocks for you to release:

The Past

While I've talked about looking at the past to understand where you are in the present, you must also paradoxically let go of the past.

Some wellbeing programmes are based on therapies that involve analysis of past events and experiences. However, let's look at this approach logically. You cannot change the past or what other people have done. What has happened has happened. A major part of the principle of letting go is releasing things beyond your control. You can analyse the past and you can analyse why people treated you a certain way, or try to understand other people's behaviour towards you and your reactions to them. But you can't ever really know whether your interpretation of events (or people's behaviour) is correct; it's merely an educated guess or a theory that you have embedded in your thoughts as real.

Who knows why past events happened and who knows why people did certain things to you. These things can certainly take up a lot of energy as you hypothesize about them, but no one has the correct answer. The uncertainty of this approach is not always helpful, especially if you reach incorrect conclusions. Interpretations are merely opinions; they are not always fact.

The other difficulty with using the past to make decisions about your present or future self is that you risk bringing emotional baggage to a situation. So, if you have a colleague who has always been difficult, or are in a relationship where someone has treated you in a way you didn't like, you start to form an opinion about them based on those experiences. This opinion might be right or might be wrong.

Certainly, if someone has caused you significant harm, it's rational to base your opinion on this – after all, you need to protect yourself. However, you may begin to adopt this attitude in every aspect of your life. The danger? You become closed to the possibility of change. When the past informs how you approach a situation, you close the door to new possibilities. As you view the present through the lens of the past, you no longer have an open mind.

One comment I often receive from people who undertake a mindfulness programme is that practising a mindful way of life affects every single aspect of their being. The core principle of mindfulness is to stay present. That means being not just physically present but also present in your emotions and your surroundings. Time and time again, you will notice that your relationships change just as a by-product of living mindfully.

Blaming Willpower

The second concept to release is willpower – the idea that somehow the reason you're not experiencing change or meaningful results in your life is because you lack willpower. This is a major block you can put upon yourself. Both mental and physical wellbeing are natural to human nature: you were born and entered the world in a state of wellbeing. So, to expect wellbeing is not some far-out idea. Our natural state is not one of stress – it's one of relaxation. This is why this wellbeing programme has been carefully formulated to work *with your body, not against it.*

If life was simple and all that was needed was willpower, then once you achieved a desired change through strong willpower you should in theory continue to sustain that willpower – because you could see that your approach has worked. But, as we know, life is not that simple. Life is messy.

Life is complicated and has many different aspects. The idea that a lack of willpower is responsible for your problems can lead you to feel only one way: like a failure. When you cannot modify your behaviour, or sustain positive changes, you start to feel guilty and worthless. You begin to think negatively about yourself and assume that if you lack willpower, you must be weak. This is neither true nor helpful. My advice is to abandon this concept altogether.

Quick Fixes

A big part of the work here in this programme is to manage expectations. Having expectations or goals that you don't meet allows those same feelings of failure and negative self-talk to start creeping in. This does most damage when you don't notice that your inner voice is talking to you this way. If this continues daily, frequently, several times a day for months on end, it will erode your very being.

One expectation I would certainly like you to let go of is that of a 'quick fix', because there's no getting around the fact that you need to do the work. Quick fixes lead to short-term results. Think about how crash diets give you instant results but then eventually the weight comes back on – in fact, often it's even more weight than you started with. It's like taking paracetamol for recurrent migraines without addressing the root problem, so the problem keeps recurring. As your guide and mentor, I want the very best for you. You deserve the very best, despite what you think.

You As the Victim

Let us talk about the victim mentality, where you are the centre of everything. The way you view yourself hugely shapes your outer reality. Adopting thoughts such as, 'Why me?' inhibits personal growth and your potential to change. You enter a state of helplessness as you put excessive focus on external factors, many of which are beyond your control. When you shift the power of control to yourself, you start to adopt a solution-focused way of life. Your mind looks for opportunities and possibilities rather than to a negative self-image where you feel at the mercy of the outside world. You begin to feel motivated to engage in self-help. The victim mentality makes one apathetic.

This is not to dismiss the great hardships and difficulties you've experienced in your life; I know that some of you have faced very significant emotional and physical pain. But I want you to gain control over the impact of those events, rather than letting them control you.

Remember, the victim mentality may be so ingrained in your psyche that you don't realize you're living this way. The heart of mindfulness is to be mindful of your thoughts and feelings. So, once again, it will take some mental retraining to notice when you have entered the victim mentality. This skill takes time, but just noticing the thoughts is a win.

Conversations Between You and Your Mind

The final practice to let go of is self-criticism. You don't realize it because you do it so often, but you have conversations with yourself hour by hour, minute by minute. Just like making the same journey in your car every morning, these conversations become automatic. You don't have to think about where to turn left or which route to take because you've done it hundreds of times. When you do something repeatedly you enter a dream-like state, where the action becomes habit. Your mind just goes into autopilot.

When the mind continually talks to you in a negative way for years and years, this becomes your natural state. You don't even notice that you're doing it. Yet the way you talk to yourself is not the way that you would ever talk to others. You cannot expect changes from a state of self-loathing. Has shaming yourself ever motivated you into sustainable action?

The next time you meet with your friends or colleagues, notice that you're very good at analysing other people. The gossip is often about who is doing what, or why they did certain things, and then you offer your opinion on it. This could be with malicious intent, or you might not mean any harm and think you're just enjoying a good discussion with those around you. However, how you treat others provides a lens on how you view yourself. Viewing others harshly and critically puts your own thoughts on a certain wavelength, and your brain becomes hardwired to look at life and yourself in that way. All this is work but the shifts are enormous. To let go of anything requires only one action: awareness.

Doctor's Prescription:
Check In

Set an hourly reminder on your phone and check in. What thoughts are you having about others and yourself? What story have you invented in your mind? How is your body physically reacting to that story – does it feel positive or negative? Most stories will not serve your wellbeing.

As soon as you are aware of negative thoughts, pause. Place a distance between you and them. Watch them go. In time, you will notice that you are more aware. The more aware you become, the less awareness is needed – because these negative thoughts are no longer a part of you.

Self-Forgiveness

A journey of self-healing must consider the ability to practise self-forgiveness. The idea of forgiving yourself is extremely powerful as it frees you from the idea of perfection. Allowing yourself to make mistakes and the freedom to grow from them, without harsh self-criticism, is essential for self-development.

In the world of science, it takes many attempts to get meaningful results. Take for example the Covid vaccines. Initially, there was the research phase, which involved laboratories around the world working to find ways to induce an effective immune response. The vaccines then underwent rigorous testing to assess safety; and this was followed by a review by regulatory bodies, which continued to monitor the vaccines' safety and efficacy. Finally, before distribution, specialist facilities were required to help manufacture and deliver the vaccine. Along the way, many mistakes were made, and many vaccines did not pass. However, this is an acceptable and normal aspect of any research. It is in this open space that learning takes place. With each unsuccessful vaccine, new knowledge was gained about what would work and what would not. There is no rebuke or criticism if setbacks occur along the timeline.

Thomas Edison made one thousand unsuccessful attempts at inventing the light bulb. When asked, 'How did it feel to fail one thousand times?' he replied, 'I didn't fail one thousand times. The light bulb was an invention with one thousand steps.' Sir James Dyson worked on 5,126 prototypes before creating a properly working vacuum and is now a worldwide household name. Behind many great inventions and success stories are countless hours, near-misses and great mistakes that led to the final outcome ...

Yet you don't allow yourself the same freedom. Rather, the default response when something doesn't go right the first time around is to give up with an air of resignation and self-criticism, labelling yourself as a failure. But we've all said or done things that we've later regretted. Sometimes we repeat this behaviour even though we know it is wrong – an unkind word or intentionally hurting someone's feelings or harming someone in some way. Despite the fact that these actions don't produce positive feelings in ourselves, the behaviour becomes addictive. Self-forgiveness provides a mechanism to promote positivity as well as to change toxic behaviour.

Leave Regret Behind

Mindfulness allows you to free yourself from the past, without replaying negative events that bring down your self-worth. Living in regret cannot lead to healing. Acknowledging and allowing for mistakes, while cultivating self-compassion, allows you to move forward. Without forgiveness, you will have failure. Without forgiveness, you will feel guilt. Without forgiveness, you will feel self-loathing.

There has been a vast amount of research into self-forgiveness. One 1992 study by Paul Mauger and colleagues showed that self-forgiveness is linked with positive emotions, high self-esteem and lower levels of anxiety and depression. A 2010 study by Michael Wohl and colleagues showed that other benefits include reducing procrastination, as demonstrated in students. Research in 1998 by Michael McCullough and colleagues also found that forgiveness acts as a driver for motivational change.

The human mind can be brutal. By replaying events and magnifying them in your own thoughts, getting you caught up in them so you feel totally engulfed, the mind thinks it is protecting you. It is in a survival mode. The mind is trying to tell you not to make the same error in the future and it does this by shaming you. But this approach rarely works. Empathy and self-forgiveness are intertwined. Thinking about others and considering their viewpoint allows you to better understand problems that arise. This doesn't mean neglecting your own needs or being passive in relationships. Forgiveness is actually a very strong tool for your own self-development and resilience. The point here is to practise self-forgiveness with yourself and with others.

Healthy Relationships

Self-forgiveness plays a fundamental role in our relationships. Whether we like it or not, we are connected to people. Part of life is interacting with others, including those online as well as in person. Even people in good financial standing have the basic need for love and union with others, a deep and meaningful connection to fulfil the human instinct of companionship.

Holding resentment towards others based on your past interactions with them can lead to problematic relationships. Unhealthy relationships can take their toll on your mental and physical wellbeing. Sometimes you won't be able to change a relationship and the other person will continue their toxic behaviour no matter how hard you try. However, for most of you, there is always hope and room for growth in your relationships. When one person enters an interaction with an open mind and brings forgiveness, releasing negative emotions, it lays the foundation to enable effective communication and ultimately a healthier relationship.

If you give others space to make mistakes and are honest and show compassion, they will inevitably start to incorporate that attitude in your relationship too. Ultimately you're creating an environment where you both feel appreciated and accepted.

Revisiting the science of the human brain, it is wired so that when you do something that makes you feel good, you get a release of dopamine, which encourages you to repeat that behaviour (the reward system). The heart of this programme is to give you the necessary frameworks to be the master of your own healing journey. This means you can use this guide to control how you deal with adverse events that happen in your life.

Negativity Bias

Your brain is also wired to be addicted to negative thoughts. This is often referred to as the negativity bias. This principle states that the mind pays more attention to negative experiences than positive ones. These experiences may be emotional or physical. It could be an unkind word, or focusing on the missing 10 per cent when you score 90 per cent in a test rather than the overwhelmingly positive result. Think about when you look at reviews before booking a holiday – a hotel might receive ninety-nine positive comments, but one damning review can alter your perception and send you looking elsewhere.

The negativity bias is thought to have been a survival mechanism. Paying attention to danger was key to prehistoric man if he wanted to live to tell the tale of being chased by predators. A 2013 study by Kelly Goldsmith and Ravi Dhar showed that negativity bias is linked to task motivation, so people are more likely to make a change based on negative feelings than they are based on positive ones. For example, the fear of being burgled will cause you to make sure you have locked the door and to check this and check again. The risk of losing something will motivate you into action more than the goal of gaining something will. However, humans in modern society no longer have the same predators and losses – despite what your brain tells you, these are rare. Yet the negativity bias phenomenon remains strong.

The problem with the negativity bias is that living in fear and dwelling on the negative events will lead you to miss the positive ones. They fly right by you. This leaves little room for positivity and happiness. Reliving negative events also puts you in a state of mind that makes those events more important than they really are and you come to believe them as 'truth'. Living with negativity bias puts you in a heightened state. Remembering that unkind word from your partner or boss will put your defences up, despite any good intentions they may have. Understanding and recognizing negativity bias is a fundamental tool on the journey of self-forgiveness and therefore self-healing.

How to Practise Self-Forgiveness

Appreciating the concept of self-forgiveness and incorporating it into your healing journey might seem unnatural at first, because we are so used to *not* living like this. So, it will take some conscious effort to begin with.

The first step is to acknowledge that you will make mistakes and that those mistakes are not linked in any way to your self-worth. Think about an event that didn't go to plan and you felt that you were to blame for that. Blame is something that we're all very familiar with. Notice the feelings that come up when you're thinking about that event. Is it making you cringe? Are there any physical feelings, such as discomfort in your abdomen or chest? Has your heart rate increased? Any sudden tension in your body, such as in your hands or jaw? Are you starting to fidget? Is your mind wanting you to think about something else? These are all signs that you are uncomfortable and are evidence of self-blame.

In a 2021 study looking at the psychological meaning of self-forgiveness, Hisn-Ping Hsu wrote that 'self-forgiveness requires a cognitive reframing of one's views of the self. It may be a positive situational strength, and it has been shown that higher levels of self-forgiveness are related to wellbeing.' He highlights that the culture and society you live in form an important aspect of self-forgiveness. For example, those in Western societies focus on the idea of the individual and personal freedom, whereas Eastern cultures emphasize the idea of people as a collective, where rules and obedience are promoted. Culture can affect self-forgiveness if acknowledging your mistakes is not seen as socially acceptable. However, in collective cultures and communities, empathy plays a more prominent role.

You need to recognize your perception and interpretation of events. A mindful practice is a wonderful way to help address this in a healthy way – and the practice called 'loving-kindness' is a particularly suitable meditation for deep healing. Jon Kabat-Zinn uses this meditation as part of his mindfulness-based stress reduction (MBSR) programme.

Another useful tool to overcome self-criticism is journalling, which allows you to explore those feelings. Many of my clients say that once they are in the flow of writing, the words just pour out onto the page without effort. Journalling allows you to extract those deep feelings, making you aware of your own thoughts about yourself. This is not something that we usually give time to but is pivotal. Ongoing mindfulness and journalling will give you the tools to foster self-forgiveness, which is also an ongoing process.

Doctor's prescription:
Positive Storytelling

Over the centuries, the thinking mind has developed to become constantly involved in storytelling, but its perception of events is often skewed because that is how the mind operates to keep you in survival mode.

Reframing the word 'mistakes' into 'learning opportunities' is probably the most important action that you can take. Write down something that you have previously thought was a mistake or that you blamed yourself for – where your recollection of the event involved a negative self-image.

Is there an alternative way you can think about that event, taking a kinder, compassionate approach to yourself?

Go through it again in your mind, as if watching it as a movie on a screen, where you are the director and the scriptwriter.

The Science of Gratitude

From the Latin word *gratia* meaning gratefulness, the psychological definition of gratitude is 'a positive emotional response that we perceive on giving or receiving a benefit from someone'. Gratitude has also been defined in some circles as the 'social glue' that strengthens human relationships, forming a pillar of society.

While practising gratitude is now quite a popular activity, it is not so easy to do. In a consumerist society, we are constantly being bombarded with messages encouraging us to buy things we 'need'. These things can be anything, from holidays to the latest gadgets to big experiences. This type of messaging focuses on the *lack* in your life rather than gratitude for what you already have.

A 2020 study by a research team for the Max Planck Institute for Evolutionary Anthropology looked at the behaviour of chimpanzees in different environments. The scientists blocked access to food so it had to be released, but the chimpanzees could choose between food for themselves and their partner or food only for them. The results demonstrated overwhelmingly that chimpanzees chose to access food for both themselves and their partner. This highlighted that the animals had an awareness of social cooperation and gratefulness. This notion is supported by the finding that chimpanzees have raised levels of the 'love' hormone oxytocin when they are cooperating with others.

There is abundant scientific research showing that practising gratitude has positive impacts on the human brain. From a biochemical point of view, it promotes the release of two neurotransmitters, dopamine and serotonin, which have a key role in making us feel happy.

Dopamine release is fast and can be triggered by a variety of things, from shopping to eating to meditating. It is known as the 'feel-good' neurotransmitter and has a role in reinforcement, which explains why one chocolate is never enough. Dopamine release also causes an intense 'high' when taking drugs such as cocaine. Its quick feel-good effect has led to it being referred to as a natural antidepressant. The role of dopamine is also significant in medical illnesses such as Parkinson's disease, which is caused by a loss of dopamine-secreting cells in the brain, and in painful conditions such as fibromyalgia, where abnormal dopamine transmission has been shown. Research has shown that undertaking activities that boost your wellbeing, such as yoga and journalling, can help release dopamine.

Serotonin levels are reduced in depression, and modern antidepressant drugs known as serotonin reuptake inhibitors (for example, Citalopram or Prozac) function by increasing the amount of serotonin available to the brain. Serotonin is also involved in the regulation of sleep, sexual health, wound healing, digestion and memory.

By regulating stress hormones such as cortisol, gratitude also has a positive impact on reducing fear and anxiety. Practising gratitude daily can help to strengthen neural pathways and create a positive feeling within yourself. This phenomenon is called *neuroplasticity* (see page 217). Gratitude can vary widely, from saying a simple thank you to buying someone a lavish gift. The same neurotransmitters are released regardless of the event.

To study the effects of gratitude on the brain, neuroscientist Glenn Fox and colleagues conducted an experiment in 2015 where gratitude was stimulated in participants while they underwent brain MRI scans. Fox found testimonies in which Holocaust survivors detailed receiving gifts or help. These were rewritten in the first person and given to participants, who pictured themselves as those survivors. Participants were then asked to put themselves in that situation and results showed increased activity in the anterior and medial cortex of the brain.

A 2009 study by Roland Zhan and colleagues found that gratitude resulted in increased grey matter in the brain. A 2012 study by psychologist Amie Gordon and colleagues showed that gratitude promotes personal relationships. These studies demonstrated that people who felt more appreciated by their partners in turn appreciated them. This also influenced the likelihood of staying in that relationship.

Practising gratitude in the workplace helps to foster bonding. Professor Sara Algoe wrote about this in *The Wall Street Journal* in 2023, outlining her research on gratitude over two decades, and her finding that employees who are grateful are more efficient and motivated, which increases productivity. She advised that people should look for opportunities to express gratitude to others, for example via email or in person, and emphasized the need to make it personal: 'we call it putting the "you" in "thank you".' Making the practice of gratitude genuine and publicly expressing thanks can have an even stronger effect on the team.

The Benefits of Gratitude

⬦ Increased resilience

⬦ Improved sleep

⬦ Pain relief

⬦ Reduced depression and anxiety

⬦ Enhanced positive thinking

⬦ Reduced negative thoughts

⬦ Increased empathy

⬦ Problem-solving

⬦ Easier forgiveness

⬦ Sustained relationships

⬦ Positive effects in cardiovascular disease and inflammatory conditions

Gratitude Writing

I like to do a gratitude list every day. I call it a gratitude list because my brain seems to be more at ease with this term than with 'gratitude journal' – which I reserve for doing self-reflection work. Both are essential daily tasks, but my gratitude list is really to give myself a quick burst of positive energy, to make me feel good. I like to write it first thing in the morning to set my day.

Like most things in this programme, this practice is dose-dependent: the more you do it, the greater the benefits. I like to count a minimum of ten things that I'm grateful for, because I think fewer than ten doesn't have the required impact and going for a minimum of ten really forces me to reflect on my day. I have never struggled to fill the list! The beauty of this simple exercise is that it really highlights the small things we often take for granted in life. In time, you will notice yourself how your thinking becomes completely rewired as you view things from a different perspective.

The benefit of gratitude writing is well known. In a 2018 study by Y. Joel Wong and colleagues, psychotherapy clients were split into three groups: one receiving psychotherapy, one assigned to psychotherapy plus expressive writing and the third group assigned to psychotherapy plus gratitude writing. Those involved in expressive writing wrote about their thoughts and feelings regarding stressful experiences. Those involved in gratitude writing wrote letters to others expressing their thanks. The study concluded that those involved in gratitude writing reported significantly better mental health than those in the other two groups.

A study in 2015 by Lea Waters and Helen Stokes found that Australian schoolchildren who kept gratitude journals had a more balanced view of the positive and negative aspects of school and experienced more positive emotions, which also helped relationships. Your list doesn't need to include major things. In fact, I would avoid concentrating on big events as you may feel there's a lack of them, which will bring your energy down.

A Sample Gratitude List

1. I am grateful for the water that comes instantly from my bathroom tap.
2. I am grateful I have a pillow at night to keep me comfortable.

3. I'm grateful to the postman who delivered my important letter.
4. I'm grateful for my laptop, which allows me to connect with other people.
5. I'm grateful for the oxygen in the air that keeps me alive.
6. I'm grateful for the satellite navigation that allowed me to get to my new destination with ease.
7. I am grateful for YouTube, which showed me a new recipe to make for dinner for my family.
8. I'm grateful for the flowers in my garden that provide nectar for the bees.
9. I am grateful for the wonderful news that my son's teacher relayed to me.
10. I am grateful for the cooker that allowed me to make a healthy breakfast this morning to help with my weight journey.

It's that simple. As you can see, this is not a time-consuming exercise. Key to completing this task successfully is being specific about people, times and other information. If you can, go into detail.

You can use any medium, be it a pen and paper, a specific gratitude diary, a quiz or an app. When you have moments of feeling particularly down, you can just revisit your list or journal for a reminder of all the positives in your life.

Doctor's Prescription:
Start Your Gratitude Journal

When we want to develop a new habit, starting is always the biggest hurdle. Once you get into the rhythm of it, it becomes second nature. Try a few prompts to get you going.

Have a think about yesterday and begin with five small things that you're grateful for, then try to build this up to ten. Alternatively, you may want to think about specific people in your life who have helped you, from the cashier at the supermarket to the Amazon delivery person, your work colleagues, or your partner. You may want to focus on specific skills or abilities, including parts of your body that enable you to do certain daily tasks.

Think about what you're doing at this moment and what provisions have allowed you to be doing it. You may wish to divide your life into different areas, such as personal and professional, and think about things you're grateful for in each.

Scripting Serenity

This book requires daily reading for a suggested duration of about twenty minutes. However, that's just a guide. Everyone's reading pace is specific to them; and sometimes you may need to re-read a paragraph several times, especially if you have a lot on your mind.

Be mindful of blindly reading information without processing it. If your mind is preoccupied, you can easily read a chunk of text and have no clue what was said. You don't have to read everything in one go; you can read in bite-size sessions of five minutes if that works better for you. Remember that this is a process of self-discovery. Throughout the journey, you will learn what works well for you and what does not. You really need to incorporate the concepts of the programme into your core beliefs.

How you read is more important than getting through the text. Reading is a skill and there is a technique to it; like everything in the programme, the more you do, the better you will be at retaining the information. Speed reading will not win any awards here. What I love about reading is its simplicity. It requires no fancy apps or tools, just your presence – and yet it has enormous power to change your life.

The Power of Reading and Writing

This may feel like going back to school, but I cannot overemphasize the importance of notetaking while reading. Again, how you do this is a personal preference; revision cards, a notebook, or your phone are all fine. Summarize the key concepts that apply to you. Do this in a way that if you were to revisit them ten years later you'd still know exactly what the information meant. So, simplify the principles and revisit them whenever you have five minutes in your day. This way, your mind will begin to accept them as real.

To be an active reader and not someone who is just passively going through the sentences, you should make reading a mindfulness practice. Keep distractions to a minimum and try not to multitask. Be in a quiet place, put any extra devices away, and have a pen and paper or your chosen notetaking device to hand. Avoid times when you are particularly tired, such as just before bed or after a heavy meal, so that you're fully alert and in a learning state. Just like when you revised for exams, don't be afraid to highlight books – write all over them, and free yourself from the idea that books need to stay in pristine condition. This is your life guide, so let it appear used. Gain a sense of accomplishment from the folded pages and annotations. It means you are doing the work.

I was privileged to be taught by the late Queen Elizabeth's personal physician, Dr Richard Thompson, who conveyed the well-known principle to medical students that to learn a key concept you need to 'See one, do one, teach one'. This is like the Feynman Technique developed by physicist Richard Feynman, a Nobel Prize winner and lecturer. He believed that with effort, anyone could learn even complicated subjects such as physics. If he lacked knowledge of a subject, he did not shy away from it; instead, he used a systematic approach to learning. He advocated a four-step process and discouraged rote learning through memorization.

The Feynman Technique

1. Identify the subject you wish to learn.
2. Write it down as if you were teaching it to someone else.
3. If you need help, go back to any sources such as books, articles, or the internet.
4. Adjust your notes if necessary, adding further explanations if needed.

Teaching something really forces you to understand a topic, which is why this technique is so powerful. It encourages you to reflect on whether you have grasped the information and in time you will gain confidence.

Note-taking is also a more active form of learning. In his 2007 study with Scellig Stone, surgeon Mark Bernstein recorded every error that he made at work over a ten-year period, from a stitch sewn incorrectly to miscommunication. This record-keeping dramatically reduced his errors, highlighting how important writing is in the learning process. Again, don't be judgemental and think that your note-keeping needs to be pretty and neat; these are your notes and you can present them however you wish. The act of writing ensures that you retain information.

Doctor's Prescription:
Pen Versus iPad?

How does the feeling of turning pages in a book compare to typing on your device? Using a laptop or the like involves fewer motor skills than a pen and paper, which is why you can lie on your bed entering information on your phone, but to write on paper you really need to be sitting at a desk. It requires more effort. Society today is all about doing things with the least effort.

But should we be more concerned with the easiest route or the best results? Writing with pen and paper is a multisensory experience, requiring visual skills and the use of touch. The action of turning pages makes a distinct sound and the release of compounds from the ink and paper produces a characteristic odour often found in new books. When you write something down, the memory of doing so becomes ingrained in the brain in a much deeper way than if you were to type it.

Writing also involves a multistep process learned in childhood: from the forming of shapes, the insertion of spaces, balancing letters on lines, to the creation of individual letters and the final step of combining those letters into words. It is a learning practice that activates different parts of the brain.

At the heart of this book is mental reprogramming to encourage you to stay present and balance your inner being. Try to incorporate physical writing in some of the elements of the programme to strengthen those neural pathways.

Meditations

Meditations for Week Two are designed to lay the foundation of your camp. With a strong base, your camp will remain stable and erect in any weather condition.

That Which Must Come to Pass

There are many events that use up your energy or that you obsess over even though you have no control over them. It is best just to leave these events in the past, without carrying their emotional toll – which will weigh you down. You can do this exercise lying down or sitting up. Settle yourself, free from any physical or mental distractions.

1. Begin by closing your eyes. Bring yourself to the present moment by focusing on your breath. As you do this, your nervous system will begin to soothe and

your heart rate will slow down.

2. Now imagine yourself standing at the edge of a lake, the water still and clear. Surrounding the lake are rocks and tall trees. The sky is a clear blue, reflecting the lake without a single cloud in sight. You can smell the fresh water and that woody fragrance of the outdoors. You hear a slight rustling of the leaves and a flock of birds flies by.

3. The water at the edge of the lake gently meets the shore. The sound of those small waves rippling by your feet brings a sense of stability and peace. A feeling of openness comes over you in this vast space, as you become receptive to whatever this moment brings.

4. You look down and notice some pebbles by your feet. You pick one up, feeling its weight in your hand and noticing its smooth surface. This pebble represents a thought that's been playing on your mind. Maybe that thought has been with you for weeks or months. Bring this worry to the forefront of your mind.

5. Now take the pebble and throw it as far as you can into the lake. 'Splash!' – it hits the water and quickly sinks to the bottom. Thoughts and feelings that have weighed you down are now at the bottom of the lake, among the many other pebbles. In fact, there are so many other pebbles that if you were to try to retrieve your worry pebble, you would not find it.

6. You may have another concern on your mind. If so, bring that one to the forefront. Pick up another pebble, let it represent that worry and then throw it into the lake. As far or as close as you wish. Throw as many pebbles as your heart desires.

7. With each throw, notice the peace and serenity that begin to fill your inner being, and the heaviness removed from your mind and your heart.

8. You feel a lightness in your shoulders now, knowing that the pebbles are at the bottom of the lake, lost forever. The pebbles, like your worries, can easily separate from your physical being. Separation just requires a simple action and awareness that they no longer need to stay where they are. You wonder how many pebbles have passed this lake over time; how many worries are now eternally lost.

9. For every difficult moment you encounter, you can take comfort in knowing every difficulty will always loosen its grip on you.

THE RANKS

There are several layers to your inner wellbeing. Ultimately, you want to reach a state of equilibrium from where you can heal – the highest rank, which you thoroughly deserve.

Take this time to allow yourself a moment of self-care.

Having a harmonious mindset between body and mind will help foster your internal balance.

Experience this equilibrium through non-attachment to your thoughts and feelings.

Recognize your internal weather pattern at this moment with kind curiosity.

Accept those thoughts and feelings with non-judgement or self-criticism.

Notice your breath to release you from the preoccupation of thoughts that keep you from the present moment.

Know that your breath is an anchor to peace and tranquillity, a state that you can access whenever you need to; it is at your daily disposal.

Sense any thoughts that draw attention away from your breath, releasing the desire to control; instead, just surrender and let things be.

The Ways of Ascent

From here, your journey is going in only one direction – upwards! This is a great meditation to use for growth and self-development.

1. Begin by finding a comfortable position in a chair, where you will stay present without falling asleep. Close your eyes and notice the point of contact between you, the chair and the floor. Start to pay attention to your breath.
2. As you settle into this meditation, begin to visualize a dense green forest, the tops of the trees swaying gently against the blue skies. You can hear the rustling of the leaves and an earthy autumn aroma catches your attention.
3. As you look up, you notice the majestic nature of the trees, which stand firmly – providing much-needed

oxygen and taking away the waste produced by the body as carbon dioxide. Regardless of the weather, the trees continue to function, paying no attention to anyone else.

4. Show gratitude to the trees that support your existence and provide inspiration; in the face of adversity, they will continue to remain tall and strong.

5. Draw strength from the forest. Its unwavering energy now has become embedded into your internal system.

6. You feel grounded, strong and secure, at one with this forest that envelops you. You feel a sense of ascension as your emotions begin to rise, just like the trees.

7. These trees have witnessed history for hundreds of years, yet they continue to grow and thrive. They do not let the past affect their core, and nor do they let the uncertain future stop them from being a stabilizing force.

8. You must also focus on the now, putting the past behind you. Don't become preoccupied with the future.

9. Take a final deep breath as you soak up the calm and stillness of the forest.

10. Conclude the meditation with a further moment of gratitude as you fill your body with refreshing and revitalizing breath that will carry you throughout your day.

Opening the Heart

The heart is the lifeforce and the very centre of your existence. This meditation will help strengthen its presence in your life as you embrace a holistic approach to wellbeing.

1. Notice if you are having a difficult moment: bring your awareness into it rather than pushing it away. We are going to facilitate this moment through the heart as well as the mind.
2. Place both hands over your heart, which will stimulate the vagus nerve. Activating this neural response will help you to feel more relaxed.
3. Notice any feelings or thoughts. Recognize any physical areas of discomfort or pain, or changes in your breathing pattern.
4. What does the mind want to do here? Does it want to think of something else? Instead of recoiling, embrace a sense of openness as you explore what is here.
5. Remind yourself that this is a safe space, a place to reflect and to grow. A place where you will learn that previous triggers in your life can be dealt with in a different way.
6. Continue to breathe into any areas of tension.
7. Are there any lingering feelings of anger, regret, guilt, concern or apprehension? Breathe into those and breathe out, letting your shoulders drop and generally feeling a lightness from head to toe.
8. Remember that whatever has happened in the past cannot be changed, but what *is* in your control is how much you let things affect your wellbeing.

9. Whatever arises, just soften into it, letting it be. You do not need to change anything at this moment, just remain present.

10. Quite quickly, you will notice that those strong feelings of discomfort have now lessened in intensity. Stay here for as long as you need to, with the breath, in the present moment.

Building the Campfire

The final step is to clear any lingering debris. Identify the difficulties in your life and use this meditation to build your camp unobstructed.

1. Set a timer so that you won't be disturbed for the next ten minutes, or whatever length of time you want to set aside.

2. Sit comfortably, relax your body, close your eyes and start to take deep breaths.

3. Imagine you are in a clearing in the centre of a forest. The air feels warm, and you take comfort from the sound of wildlife and a stream flowing nearby. As you gaze up, you notice the sun streaming through the canopy onto your hands.

4. You look at some branches on the ground by your feet. Now, without self-criticism or judgement, recall all the challenges you're facing. Each of those branches represents a difficulty.

5. Place the branches one by one into the centre of a clearing. You may wish to name them as you go along. 'This one represents my project deadline'; 'This one

concerns the money difficulties I have'; 'This branch is my relationship' and so forth.

6. You notice two flintstones. You strike them together, creating a spark that you use to light the branches, creating a small fire.

7. At first, the fire is a shock as it lights quickly and spreads throughout the branches.

8. But then you notice a sense of comfort, because the fire is well-contained and provides warmth. It is not as frightening as you thought.

9. Soon the fire settles, as there are no branches left. At this moment, affirm to yourself: 'I am resilient. I have faced my challenges head-on and now I'm ready to move on with my life.'

10. There remain only ashes now where the fire once stood. You realize that the challenges you feared were not as bad as you had imagined.

Informal Mindfulness Practice

Reflect on This Week

We doctors are taught to reflect on our experiences as part of our job. In fact, reflection is a prerequisite to keeping our medical licence from the General Medical Council. Reflection is encouraged in many professions. Its power is enormous – it helps you to learn from mistakes, to try something different and to connect with yourself. Here, I recommend a simple method that is easy to engage with, so that you'll be sure to repeat it often.

Recall a practice or skill that you did this week. Then ask yourself the following questions and write the answers down:

- ◇ What went well?
- ◇ How did it make you feel?
- ◇ Did you notice any changes in your life, however small?
- ◇ What could you have improved on?

Mindful Eating

Suggested time: ten minutes daily.

Choose one meal. Sit without distractions – put away your phone and other devices. You want to be fully present and engage all your senses to develop the art of mindfulness.

1. Notice your whole body – where it is in contact with the chair, the floor, and the table. Notice the cutlery you're using. Examine each utensil as if you're seeing it for the first time.
2. Like any mindfulness practice, your mind will wander. Let it, and bring it back gently to your meal.
3. Pick up an item of food. Notice its shape, size and colours. Engage other senses, appreciating its aroma; your mouth may start to water with appreciation.
4. Now take small bites, noticing the texture, the movements of the teeth and tongue to help you digest it.
5. Savour the experience with gratitude for the food and those who helped to bring it you.
6. Repeat with the next bite and notice the sensation of beginning to feel full. This might be a feeling you have dissociated from if you're struggling with weight gain. You want to notice the start of feeling full, not that bloated feeling.

END OF WEEK TWO

By the end of this week, you will have begun to gain a connection with parts of your inner being that have been neglected. You have begun to incorporate compassion and brought the heart into your daily life. By doing this, along with the practice of letting go and gratitude, you have paved the path for progress.

WEEK THREE:

MASTERING THE MIND

Now you've laid the foundation for your CAMPS, you are ready to build. The framework, the material, the essence of it all is in mindfulness. You will learn how to ground yourself with the principles of mindfulness and develop your resilience and inner strength. Like the campfire, meditation practices will supply the light, illuminating your path along the way.

Here are some skills that you will learn
to cultivate this week:

**Incorporating mindfulness
as a daily practice**

Befriending yourself

Managing difficult situations

**Understanding how mindfulness
works to ensure emotional and
mental alignment with the programme**

Starting a Mindful Way of Living

Any self-care or wellness programme that suggests you just need to show up and your life will change is making false claims. You cannot expect lasting changes to your life without work. I don't mean the nine-to-five types of work. I'm talking about a few minutes a day that you build on alongside your life's demands. Here are my top takeaways for adopting a mindful way of life ...

Forget the All-or-Nothing Rule

If this programme was hard to follow, you would check out both mentally and physically before long. When GPs like me put patients on a new drug, we start off low and slow and monitor them to see how they're tolerating it. We may adjust the dose until we find the correct one, because each patient has a dosage that suits them. Likewise, this programme is for everyone but can be tailored to your life circumstances, your goals and your motivations. Little and often is absolutely going to make changes. Try to do the activities most days if not every day.

Watch Out for Self-Sabotage

In Greek mythology, the Sirens were striking creatures with the body of a bird and the head of a human. They had captivating voices that would tempt sailors from their boats to later shipwreck them. Your self-sabotage is like the Sirens – it tempts you and you're lured by it thinking it's there for your own protection. But that's simply a trick your mind has fallen for. The likelihood is that you've been tricked like this for many years and haven't noticed.

Self-sabotage, like the Sirens, is destructive. It reinforces the negative behaviours that stand in the way of you and your success, so that you'll fall short of the goals you've set. This leads to further negativity in feelings of shame, guilt and frustration.

The Sirens were powerful but they had a weakness: if anyone heard them and survived, they perished. According to mythology, Odysseus did just that and the Sirens committed suicide by hurling themselves against rocks. Self-awareness is the Odysseus to your self-sabotage –the cornerstone of mindfulness. When you recognize a behaviour as self-sabotage, you will come to gain a dislike for it. To begin practising self-awareness means shifting out of autopilot and stopping self-sabotage in its tracks.

Self-sabotage is your enemy – the internal chatter that tries to put you off when you're trying something new. Watch out for those self-sabotaging thoughts: 'This isn't working'; 'This is silly'; 'I give up, this is my life and I should just accept it ...'

This is the mind doing what it does best. Entering an analytical, self-defensive fighting mode. It has a new opponent and doesn't know to react. You have been thinking and doing things in a particular way for many years and suddenly you're teaching your brain a new way of doing and thinking. You didn't think it was going to take that lying down?

Interpretation is Just an Opinion

Most negative thoughts are caused by irrational ideas. For example, imagine you enter your boss's office and they're immediately rude to you and tell you to get out. You promptly leave, likely feeling angry and hurt because they clearly don't like you. However, five minutes before you walked into their office, your boss received some devastating news about a member of his family and was feeling upset when you arrived. But our minds are used to processing events in a negative way because we think of ourselves as unworthy. Our interpretations of events such as this fits in with how we view ourselves.

Conversely, someone who has an abundance of confidence and self-esteem would take a period of reflection and interpret the same event in a different way. They may say to themselves that their boss's behaviour is out of character and wonder what's happened. They might give them some space and then go and ask them about it. The boss could then confirm what had happened and have the opportunity to apologize for their outburst.

Your mind is powerful. You are in control of the way you feel. You can choose how you interpret events. Of course, it may be that your boss is generally unreasonable and antagonistic. But the person who bathes in low self-esteem will go home and have lingering thoughts about that event. The person who has negative thoughts will carry those feelings of hurt and anger and may take them out on their own nearest and dearest. Perhaps at dinner their thoughts would be so consumed by the event that they couldn't focus or engage in conversation. They might be physically present, but be mentally somewhere else.

False Protection Mechanism

As Jon Kabat-Zinn says, 'You can't stop the waves, but you can learn to surf.' Remember to allow yourself time to challenge your negative thoughts with positive ones. Any programme that promises instant results is promising you a false ideal. Even the most experienced meditator has moments of difficulty. But don't see this in terms of failure; instead, free yourself from labels, because labels won't help you progress. This programme does not promise that you will never face a difficult moment again; rather, it suggests that difficult moments won't be as difficult as they once were. Your reaction to difficult moments will change.

Negative thoughts will come – this is part of human behaviour. But when you notice them, release them as if they are helium balloons. We aren't trying to pop the balloons; we're simply accepting that they're here now. Rather than waste energy trying to destroy them, just watch them float by. Remember that different people think all sorts of things and not all those things are true. Likewise, something isn't so just because a significant number of people believe it to be – how many once claimed that the Earth was flat and not round?

Don't Forget to Befriend Yourself

I often notice that the way I speak to my friends is very different to the way I speak to my family. There's a certain harshness and directness when I'm speaking to my own household. And this doesn't mean that I love my family less than I love my friends – in fact, they mean the most to me. This way of addressing them comes from familiarity and certainty. I don't need to impress them or pamper them. I know that they will still be here tomorrow. But we tend to work more on other relationships and friendships because these can come and go. As such, we're often more polite and soft with our friends, and may even go out of our way to make sure they stay in our lives.

So how about the relationship we have with ourselves? How do you talk to yourself? In much the same way, you know you're not going anywhere; you're stuck with this body and this mind forever. There's likely the same harshness and directness in how you speak to yourself. In fact, you're probably the most critical person you face every day. There's probably a constant commentary about the way you look, the way you speak ... Do you do this to anyone else?

What if you changed the way you view yourself? What if you began to view yourself as a very important person? This surely would cultivate feelings of compassion and patience. If a baby makes mistakes, you give them space to learn and grow; you don't abandon them or criticize them harshly. From now on, I want you to think of yourself as a dignitary. Someone worthy. Allow yourself time to change. This is not an overnight fix; you need to give yourself patience.

Pretend for just a few seconds that you're walking down the hallway of Buckingham Palace in London. You would walk with your back upright, your head high and your eyes looking ahead, not at the floor, because the situation has an air of dignity and respect. If you can carry yourself in this way most of the time, your feelings about yourself will start to evolve. You will leave the place where you saw yourself as unworthy of love and affection and move to a place where you are a dignitary deserving of wonderful things.

Logic Does Not Make It True

The famous neurologist Sigmund Freud had an idea that we have both a conscious mind and an unconscious mind. The conscious part of our brain is aware of our surroundings and internal environment, and of what's going on in our heads. The subconscious part of our brain is not so aware. Often, painful or unwanted thoughts are hidden away in the subconscious so we can avoid dealing with them. Furthermore, Freud suggested that our actions reflect what's going on in our minds – and that how we act is a representation of the kind of person we are. While this theory makes sense, something about it doesn't ring true.

Indeed, many psychologists and medics disagree with this concept and dispute the idea that we are our thoughts. Thoughts are not real or fact, and can change easily from moment to moment. Take the earlier example of the visit to your boss: we make interpretations based on limited information and those interpretations are not always accurate, though we take them to be real. What's more, the average person can have up to 60,000 thoughts a day, but they don't act on all of them.

Thoughts do not define us. Rather, thoughts are a response, and we can choose whether that response is positive or negative. Your thoughts have as much power as you allow them to have. The more attention you give to a thought, and the more you get caught up in it, the bigger it will become, until eventually it forms part of your identity.

Distancing yourself from your thoughts is a powerful

and simple tool to live a peaceful life. Just like self-sabotage, overthinking and getting caught up in your thoughts is destructive. You can soon become overwhelmed by them and this can manifest in physical sensations, such as headaches, pain and raised blood pressure, as well as mental symptoms, such as anxiety and depression.

Putting distance between yourself and your thoughts allows you to manage your negative ideas about the past and your procrastinations about the future. This is a central tenet of mindfulness: staying in the present moment. Just as awareness is the Odysseus to self-sabotage, mindfulness is the tool for overthinking. Recognize when you are on that train, caught up in your thoughts and unable to get off. If this is what you're doing, you'll miss new experiences in your life. For example, you may be on a holiday or in a spa but your thoughts are caught up in a previous negative event, and before you know it the holiday or deep-tissue massage is over. So, an activity you paid a lot of money for hasn't relaxed you as you'd hoped it would, because you have allowed your thoughts to be in control and have not freed yourself from them.

Doctor's Prescription:
Avoid Jumping to Conclusions

Discard the concept that an apparent correlation between two things means that one thing caused the other. Dr Franz Messerli, a cardiologist in New York, made an amusing comment in 2012, noting that countries whose population consumed a lot of chocolate also had a large number of Nobel Prize winners. The media unwittingly ran with this story as though one caused the other. But the logic was simple: developed, rich nations have more money, which results in better education, more research and luxuries like chocolate!

If you believe you will never make progress because you've already tried something and it didn't work, you have made a misinterpretation. You're adding things together and forming an incorrect conclusion. If humans all believed that change is impossible, civilization would never have progressed.

The lesson here is not to give up straightaway. Don't throw in the towel after a few attempts. Growth takes time; keep watering the plant, and given the right conditions it will grow.

Evidence and Benefits
of Mindfulness

While science is the foundation to prove concepts in the modern world, I find most of my patients do not want to be bombarded with excess scientific literature. My job is to provide a treatment plan based on the latest medical evidence; to break down complex science and convey it to my patients in a simple and comprehensive way. In this section, I will go through this process for mindfulness, presenting the evidence as though you were in my consulting room. If you would like to delve further into the scientific literature of mindfulness, I would recommend looking into the work of Jon Kabat-Zinn and Dr Mark Williams. But for the purposes of this book, I'm going to keep it simple.

Much of the science of mindfulness can be attributed to the work of Jon Kabat-Zinn and his Stress Reduction Clinic at the University of Massachusetts Medical Center during the 1980s.

His MBSR programme helped patients cope with stress and pain. The aim of this course was to promote greater self-awareness, to give people an understanding of how they react to stress so they could develop the skills to cope with stressful situations. The programme combined mindfulness meditation and yoga using the mind–body interaction.

He measured the outcomes of mindfulness in a scientific way to prove its benefits, making it acceptable to the modern world. Although initially used for hospital patients, the MBSR programme has now become the cornerstone for many and has provided a catalyst for further research into mindfulness-based interventions. There are three key components to the MBSR programme, all of which I strongly advise you to adopt:

1. To not view the practice of mindful living as something you must do for wellbeing; instead, embrace it as an opportunity and 'an adventure of living'.
2. Willingness and effort are required throughout the programme, so that participants regularly practice meditation regardless of their feelings about it on any given day.
3. Commitment is paramount, as participants must be willing to accept that there will be a lifestyle change from the outset.

The website of the renowned NHS Guy's and St Thomas' hospital in London states that MBSR can help with conditions such as chronic pain, stress and anxiety, sleep problems and daytime tiredness. It can also help with headaches, migraines, irritable bowel syndrome and dizziness and syncope.

The site advocates mindfulness for people suffering from

distressing symptoms or difficult life events, as well as those experiencing ongoing stress, such as work-related stress. The UK's National Institute for Health and Care Excellence (NICE), which provides guidance for health practitioners on evidence-based medical treatments, also advises that mindfulness can prevent relapse in depression.

Transformation in the Brain

According to 2011 research from the Harvard Medical School, brain scans have verified that structural changes in the brain occur in those who regularly practise mindfulness meditation. Measurable changes have been found in three areas of the brain:

1. Amygdala – the stress centre
2. Hippocampus – related to memory and learning
3. Prefrontal cortex – involved with decision-making

It was found that patients who underwent the MBSR programme had decreased volume in their amygdala, which is responsible for stress and anxiety. There was also thicker grey matter found in the hippocampus, which is involved in muscle control and sensory awareness. There is some thought that the loss of grey matter associated with ageing could be positively affected by meditation. It may play a part in slowing down cognitive decline in the elderly, but ongoing research is needed.

In a 2021 study looking at mindfulness-based interventions for college students, Brandon Smit and Euthemia Stavrulaki observed the effects of mindfulness meditation in the reading section of students' graduate record examinations. Students reported that their ability to recall and focus was much improved, as was reflected in their improved academic scores. Further studies using brain scans have shown less mind wandering and more stability in the ventral cortex in people who meditate.

Mark Williams and MBSR

Oxford University Professor Dr Mark Williams built on the principles of MBSR, as well as Bernard and Teasdale's concept of the 'doing' and 'being' modes, and established a mindfulness-based cognitive therapy (MBCT) for depression. Dr Williams's work was also groundbreaking. He was able to show that MBCT reduced rates of relapse in patients who suffered from recurrent depression. The programme encourages the being mode because it is in this space that emotional wellbeing can occur, especially for those who have recurrent depression.

Furthermore, research showed that the beneficial effects of MBCT led to patients on antidepressant medication being able to reduce their dose. These effects were found to last over six months in some cases. The MBCT programme centres on acceptance of one's feelings and being in the present moment. Students learn to recognize their thoughts and feelings without getting caught up in them, so they become liberated from repeated negative patterns. By creating distance between thoughts and the self, MCBT promotes positive thinking. Patients learn the tools needed to combat symptoms of depression, and can use these whenever they're faced with a difficult situation in the future.

Monkey Mind

The popular term 'monkey mind' refers to that feeling of being distracted and caught up in your own internal conversations. The idea of monkey mind was first described over 2,000 years ago by Buddha, who spoke about the human mind as being full of drunk monkeys chattering and fighting, causing a state of mental instability. As you live your modern life in constant doing mode, instead of in being mode, and are bombarded with daily digital distractions, the monkey mind is as busy as it has ever been.

The part of the brain called the default mode network (DMN) is responsible for the monkey mind. Those who suffer from an active DMN will often have wandering thoughts about the past or the future, which results in feeling overwhelmed and distracted. A 2011 study by Judson Brewer and colleagues found that those who practised mindful meditation had decreased activity in the DMN. The monkey brain then quietens down, leading to clarity of thought and decreased stress and anxiety.

Medical conditions where stress is a contributing factor, such as chronic disease and illness, eating disorders, pain, blood pressure, gastrointestinal disorders (including irritable bowel disease), fibromyalgia, panic attacks, post-traumatic stress disorder, skin disorders and insomnia, can benefit from mindfulness.

What's more, the cognitive benefits of mindfulness also include improved attention and concentration, better emotional regulation, greater adaptability, improved decision-making, memory and learning skills and decreased mind-wandering. The emotional benefits include reduced negative thinking and improved self-esteem and self-awareness, as well as fostering empathy and compassion and better ability to cope with life's challenges, such as work, family life, financial stress, or sudden changes or difficulties, including grief.

The Therapeutics of Journalling

Journalling has widespread benefits. Similarly to offloading or venting to a friend or colleague, it allows you to deal with emotions and process events. The beauty of journalling is that it allows a healthy expression of your thoughts and feelings. It can be done anywhere, anytime. This will have a ripple effect on other aspects of your life, such as focus, concentration, memory, sleep and managing stress.

This type of record-keeping can also identify negative aspects of your life. You will notice a pattern – certain events or people that evoke a strong reaction in you. Just writing these observations down can have a positive effect. It allows acknowledgement and acceptance rather than hiding or avoidance, which do not work to help with problems.

Avoidance as Protection

Avoidance behaviour is a common coping mechanism used by many. Often, we look for distractions, which can range from recreational activities such as gaming or sports to food, alcohol and socializing. Avoidance is understandable. However, it's a tactic that means we don't confront distressing and uncomfortable situations and is easy to enforce.

The purpose of avoidance is self-protection, but it can leave you feeling more anxious and stressed. Avoidance can have an impact on your personal relationships and deny you of opportunities. Journalling allows you to process events openly. It is a safe, non-confrontational space of non-judgement and openness. From here, you can start to heal. You can replace the negative self-talk and allow yourself to build healthy coping mechanisms, using all your inner tools without reliance on external factors.

Thought-Stopping

While journalling, you may feel a mix of emotions as you recall events. A common approach in dealing with this is 'thought-stopping', which can be useful if you have repeated negative thoughts. Thought-stopping is when you become aware of a thought and you acknowledge it as unwanted and decide to remove it from your consciousness. Formal thought-stopping techniques include clapping loudly or wearing a rubber band on your wrist that you pull to 'stop' the thoughts. However, research suggests that thought-stopping isn't always the best coping strategy, because it is a temporary solution and can make you have more thoughts about whatever it is you were thinking about. This is called the 'rebound effect'.

Psychologist Daniel Wegner and colleagues demonstrated this effectively in their 1987 study looking at the effects of thought suppression. He asked participants to form two groups. He asked one group to stop thinking about white bears and asked the other group to do the opposite and think about white bears. Participants in group one were instructed to be aware of anything that came to mind during the next five minutes; if they thought of a white bear, they were to ring a bell. Sure enough, they thought about white bears.

For the second part of the experiment, Wegner asked group one to do the opposite – to purposefully think about the white bears. This time, it was noted that participants thought more about white bears than participants in the second group did, despite the second group being asked to think about white bears throughout the experiment. Wegner concluded that when you make the intention to avoid a certain thought, one part of your brain enforces this while another part of your brain must make sure the unwanted thoughts stay away – and ironically, to do this it has to think about the thought that's meant to be avoided.

This is often why diets don't work: because when you try to avoid certain food groups, such as cake and biscuits, and label them as 'bad', you often find yourself thinking about them even more. Consequently, you feel like a failure for giving in, when in reality thought-stopping or avoidance are simply not practical coping strategies. Your food intake is likely to be the result of emotional eating and these approaches do not address the root cause.

How to Start Journalling

In a 2005 study looking at the benefits of expressive writing, Karen A. Baikie and Kay Wilhelm asked participants to write about events in their lives for about fifteen minutes on separate occasions. It was found that those who did this activity had better physical and psychological outcomes. The report concluded that writing can be used as a possible therapeutic tool in psychiatric conditions.

If journalling appears a daunting task, you could use prompts to get you going:

⬦ Your current goals (personal, professional).

⬦ Things you want to improve (that are in your control).

⬦ Reflection on interactions or events of the day.

⬦ Your thoughts on frustrations or blocks in your life.

You can use a laptop or just a simple notepad – journals don't have to be expensive, but if having a special book makes you feel better, then do it. Whatever works for you. I like journalling on a computer so I can go back and find keywords easily. Also, being a doctor, I find it difficult to read my own handwriting!

In a small US study in 2019, Oliver Glass and colleagues observed the outcomes of patients who had a history of trauma and undertook a short expressive-writing course, which included mindful writing prompts. The study concluded that participants showed increased resilience, decreased depressive symptoms and rumination. This is because practising journalling allows you to focus on the present moment.

When do you feel most overwhelmed or stressed? Mornings, mid-morning, evenings? This is actually a good time to journal.

Some of my clients feel journalling is a great way to unwind before going to sleep, so the mind is not overactive with replaying events or thinking about tomorrow. Alternatively, you might do it after waking up in the morning. It can be a ten-minute activity or a thirty-minute activity; there's no strict timing to follow.

Doctor's prescription:
Effective Journalling

○ Write every day, even if your day was 'insignificant' – consistency is key.

○ You're not writing an essay. Keep it simple and don't feel the need for it to be impressive.

○ There is no right or wrong way to journal – some days you may want to write pages, and at other times just a few lines.

○ Start by creating a space and time to acknowledge your thoughts and feelings.

○ Write as if no one will ever read it: knowing it's completely private will allow you to be open and honest.

o   Review your journals and notice any patterns.

o   If you are not comfortable writing, use images or
    pictures that resonate with how you're feeling.

o   I recommend keeping a separate gratitude journal
    in addition to a reflective journal.

Incorporating Silence and Solitude

Have you ever experienced silence? And I don't mean the simple absence of external noise – I mean the deep, meaningful kind of silence. The absence of thoughts swimming in your mind coupled with a peaceful and calm surrounding. Silence can be thought of as a physical entity, but it is also a state of being. It can foster a space for healing, recovery and growth.

In this space, you can truly apply the fundamental principle of mindfulness, which is awareness. Without distraction, your senses are sharpened to the visual and auditory clues of the world that you live in. In this state, you can fully appreciate the joys of life and the daily abundance that you may not appreciate. In silence, you have the ability to discover yourself. Reflection will flow so much more easily. In silence, you have the privilege of letting go and really being your true self. Silence is a powerful tool, but it is not valued.

Silence Versus Success

There is a commonly perpetuated belief that productivity means success. That we should be 'busy' and always doing something, that being productive is something to celebrate. Yet we also acknowledge that mental-health problems are on the increase, as many feel overwhelmed, burned out, stressed ... the symptoms of this 'productive' way of life. Silence is not something that is propagated. In fact, the opposite is true: silence does not fit in with the concept of productivity.

But it is in silence that we alleviate stress and allow our inner self to heal. It is in silence that we can calm our nervous system, which will foster resilience, concentration, and focus – ironically, the very tools we need to be productive.

In today's celebrity world, being socially busy is also considered a measure of success. Being surrounded by people, at parties, involved in promoting products and having an online presence are all highly revered. If you're not out on a Saturday night or celebrating an occasion such as Christmas or Halloween with a group of people, this is interpreted as some sort of failure. Such events cannot possibly be spent in silence or solitude, because these states of being are looked down upon in modern culture.

In your own life, if you don't have a large social circle – especially one that you can show on social media – or if you're not out or busy being productive, you too will have feelings of inadequacy. But our self-worth should not be linked in any shape or form to how 'busy' our lives are.

Today silence is equated with boredom, which also has negative connotations. To be silent or bored or to have nothing to do are not encouraged. Even if we're resting, we scroll on phones or channel hop, never truly being in a restful state, a silent state.

In the digital world, our attention is constantly being directed elsewhere. Distraction has become a common tool to deal with problems instead of facing them. This may seem easier. However, taking this approach means that life will remain unfulfilling. Distraction does not allow introspection, which is a pivotal tool for self-growth.

If we are uncomfortable with silence and solitude, we will often seek noise. If we start to reframe silence as stillness, though, those walls start to come down. Who doesn't like to gain a tranquil state, one of calm and stillness? Just to rest from the busyness of life, from all its demands? In work meetings we like to have minimal background noise, because it's almost impossible to focus when multiple people are talking at once. Similarly, when multiple children are talking to you at the same time it is difficult to comprehend anything that's being said.

Have you ever tried talking to someone while they're busy scrolling on their phone? Did you get frustrated and feel they weren't listening? In much the same way, having a meaningful conversation with yourself requires your complete attention. Yet instead of engaging in a truly restful state with silence when you have a moment to yourself, you start to feel guilt, thinking that you should 'busy' yourself.

Think of all the times you've experienced an enforced quiet environment. During exams, for example, silence is required to maximize your focus and concentration; in cinemas or theatres, or during music recitals, silence is needed to maximize your enjoyment. We usually prefer quiet when we go to sleep, too, and that is when the body regenerates and is restored. A 2015 study by Staci Wendt and colleagues looking at meditation in schools found that a fifteen-minute period of silence increased resilience and reduced anxiety. Participants who undertook the practice also reported better sleep, and feeling happier and more confident.

The State of Rushing

Another default mode related to busyness is rushing. We feel the need to get things done quickly because there is always more to do. Have you ever noticed the constant deadlines and targets you live with causing tension in your body, or suddenly overwhelming your mind? In the state of rushing, your mind loses clarity. The details of the task are diluted as you become preoccupied with the concept of time.

No doubt there are times you need to rush, but this should not be *all* the time. Every moment of rushing activates your sympathetic nervous system, releasing stress hormones such as cortisol and consequently elevating your blood pressure and heart rate. It is well known that increased blood pressure damages your arteries, which can lead to adverse effects on major organs such as the kidney, heart and brain.

You do not need expensive retreats and spas to experience stillness; you can create it in your own home. With the tools of visualization, your mind will believe whatever you tell it. Silence plays a fundamental role in meditation, especially in the practice of meditation. In meditative practices, you free yourself from the noise of your inner thoughts.

Doctor's Prescription:
Find Time for Silence

Start to befriend the only stability in your life: you.

- Set aside a time to immerse yourself in silence and solitude.

- Find a quiet space where you will not be disturbed.

- Put away any devices.

- You can choose to engage in an activity, such as meditating or journalling, or just sit in silence.

- Remain present.

At first this will feel uncomfortable, because you are used to doing rather than being.

Navigating Internal Storms

It is known that emotions drive events in our lives and determine their outcomes. The first step to dealing with your emotions is to recognize them. People often become so used to their emotions that they become ingrained in their personality, without them realizing they are acting a certain way.

There may be times when you get so caught up with yourself, your own thoughts and feelings, that you have no concern for those around you. During these times, your emotions seem beyond your control and they escalate rapidly, leading you to behave in ways that have repercussions for you and others. But we have all weathered our internal storms sometimes.

The exercise of acknowledging the weather pattern inside you is not designed to make you feel guilty or indulge in self-loathing. Its purpose is to help you gain control. Through practices like journalling, you can start to notice your internal storm patterns. For instance, there may be people or events that repeatedly trigger you.

The life-inventory exercise at the beginning of the book (see page 30) will also help identify sources of stress. This could be from work, home or family or stress that you have placed upon yourself. Have you set any goals that you're finding unmanageable or perhaps unrealistic? Do you have some unmet needs that are causing frustration? Maybe there are unmet needs that other people have placed upon you. I often see this in patients who are carers or have dependents. Such patients often feel a constant state of disappointment. This exercise requires some introspection and may be uncomfortable, especially if the source of stress includes past trauma. In some cases it may be advisable to do this work with a trained therapist.

Emotional Intelligence

Given that the essence of mindfulness is to stay in the present moment, it may seem strange that I'm advocating for exploration of the past. However, if your past is commonly your present then we do need to address this. Doing so will also help you develop emotional intelligence so that you can respond to situations in a healthy way, rather than reacting to them habitually. The idea of emotional intelligence has grown in popularity and involves identifying and interpreting your emotions and then managing them constructively. Emotional intelligence requires an awareness of personal strengths and limitations, which will help you to navigate any unrealistic expectations you have placed on yourself. It also involves an ability to accept change, which fosters self-confidence and leaves you better equipped to face difficult situations.

A big part of emotional intelligence is thinking about others. This is why it has become standard in many school curriculums;

it promotes thinking about how other people may feel and being able to empathize with them. Adopting this approach greatly improves communication. Any wellbeing programme must acknowledge that you are not alone in your journey; that your life involves relationships. These relationships may be fleeting or deeply meaningful, but we are all connected to someone in some way. It could be the postman who delivers your letters and parcels, the gardener who prunes your roses, or more permanent relationships, such as those with your partner, your children, your parents or work colleagues. It has been shown that those with lower emotional intelligence skills are more argumentative and have poor relationships.

A 2022 study by Lakesha Butler and colleagues looked at evidence and strategies for emotional intelligence in American pharmacy students. It found that emotional intelligence was essential in relationships and stress management, including in the self-regulation of behaviour. The study also found increasing evidence that emotional intelligence can contribute to academic success, patient care, greater life satisfaction and positive mental-health. People with higher emotional intelligence displayed strong interpersonal skills, which helps in workplace settings. Here, being able to manage your emotions, make clear decisions and work effectively within a team by developing greater empathy are all beneficial. Knowing your limitations also allows you to identify areas in the workplace you need to work on.

As should be clear by now, tools that involve mental strategies are required to navigate your inner storm when your emotions drive your actions. At the heart of this will be mindfulness and meditation, which allow you to focus on the present moment, freeing yourself from the past and concerns about the future while allowing a safe space to acknowledge how you're feeling. This can be supplemented with journalling and positive affirmations.

You will inevitably come across roadblocks on your journey through life. Rather than feeling frustrated or overwhelmed by these roadblocks, engaging with this programme will show you a way around them and help you to develop resilience as you go. Instead of adopting the victim mentality – 'Why does this always happen to me?' – you can reframe difficult events as opportunities for learning and growth. Gratitude is a key skill that will help you overcome your tendency to take a negative view and avoid downward spirals into feeling anxious or depressed. Noticing the positive events in your life, whether small or big, will enhance your coping mechanisms as you begin to view the world differently.

Doctor's Prescription:
Celebrate the Small Wins

When you notice the progress you're making, it is human nature to repeat the actions that led to it. This strengthens your emotional state, increasing your motivation. Learning to celebrate small wins is key to attaining your goals and enhancing your emotional intelligence.

Celebrating the small wins in life is also much more achievable than focusing solely on larger goals. Each small step will eventually lead to your greater goal. Concentrating on small gains will immediately boost your confidence.

Write down any small wins you have had this week. Don't forget to acknowledge the progress you've made, because incremental changes can manifest into long-lasting change. It's about having patience and perseverance. For example, you may be able to run five more minutes than you could yesterday; or you may not have lost weight but had one less biscuit; you might not have finished that project but you've written two more pages.

Meditations

Meditations for Week Three are designed to strengthen the concept of freeing yourself from the internal narration that accompanies you everywhere. You will start to bring peace and serenity through awareness and presence, the foundations of mindfulness.

Your Past, Your Future, Your Present

Often we live with a constant background chatter made up of our obsessive thinking about the past and the conversations and events we replay in our heads. The mind is also preoccupied with predicting and planning the future. These ruminations take your focus away from the present moment and ultimately your wellbeing.

1. Healing occurs in the here moment, so spend time intentionally now with your breath and your body, focusing your attention on your thoughts.

2. If there's something specific on your mind, bring your awareness to it but in a non-attached way so you are not getting caught up in the story.

3. Now see the event as a movie playing on a cinema screen, where you are not in the movie but are watching it from a distance.

4. First, bring to this movie any events in the past that have lingered in your thoughts and consumed you.

5. Let the scenes play out as you continue to observe them without judgement. Remind yourself that whatever's happened in the past cannot be undone; so, as this part of the movie finishes, it is no longer with you.

6. Now visualize any upcoming events that are making you anxious. You are the director of the movie, so you are in control of how the movie plays out in a positive way.

7. Bring a smile to your face, knowing that you no longer need to worry about future preoccupations.

8. Your movie now comes to an end. Take a deep breath and slowly exhale, opening your eyes and feeling a sense of peace because worries about the past and fears of the future no longer take centre stage in your mind.

The Monkey

There are moments when you're away from the hustle and bustle of life, recuperating and relaxing, on holiday, or in a spa, or just asleep in your bed. However, your inner voice – that monkey chatter – does not allow you to find inner peace. Learn to tame it.

1. Begin your meditation as you usually do, closing your eyes and turning your attention to your breath.
2. As you breathe out, begin to take notice of the internal dialogue that you often use to make decisions and that determines how you feel.
3. Now visualize a monkey on your shoulder. It is this monkey you have conversations with.
4. Bring to mind any recent conversations you've had with the monkey, who is separate from you but vies for and feeds on your attention.
5. What is the monkey telling you at the moment? What's on its mind? Do not try to push it away; instead, with kindness and patience, just notice the narration that it wants you to believe is real.
6. Its story could be something uncomfortable or that causes concern. Notice how this makes you feel. Are there any areas of tension or tightness?
7. Use your breath to breathe deeply into those areas. Imagine the breath as a soothing light, calming you and then calming the monkey.
8. The monkey stays with you but is content, and grateful for the kindness and attention you have shown. Whatever stories it wished to put into your thoughts remain with the monkey but are no longer part of you.
9. Appreciate the quietness, a space of tranquillity. You can return here whenever the monkey requires your attention.

The Olive Tree

The olive tree dates to Ancient Greek mythology as a symbol of peace. This is a quality that every human would wish to achieve in their life: peace with others, and peace with themselves.

1. Close your eyes and sit up, with the crown of your head tilted a little towards the sky. Relax your shoulders, soften your belly and begin to breathe in and out.
2. As you sit, start to pay attention to your breath and notice that the mind will try to involve itself as thoughts. Let it, but observe the thoughts and watch them go by.
3. In between those thoughts, there will be moments when you are paying full attention to the breath. It is in these moments of stillness that there is peace.
4. Imagine you are the tall tower of an olive tree, firmly rooted in the ground, drawing nourishment from the soil where it is planted.
5. Your potential is like the branches that reach out to the sky; there is no limit. The only resources you need are the sun and the air, which belong to no one but are there whenever you need them.
6. The thoughts that hold you back are represented by wilted leaves that naturally fall to the ground.
7. The vibrant, strong, green leaves high up on the tree are thoughts that strengthen you and continue to shape you in a positive direction. You are the sturdy trunk. You are strong and present.
8. Now take those feelings and let them provide you with a stabilizing force throughout your day.

The Master

Being able to process feelings such as anger and resentment will free up a lot of wasted energy and reduce anxiety, improving your self-esteem. Anger is a natural defence to cope with situations, your mind hoping that it will improve it. Bringing mindfulness to anger ensures that you acknowledge it but manage it in a healthy way.

1. Sit in a quiet space, close your eyes to eliminate any distractions and gently sense any underlying emotions in your mind or body. Acknowledge them and remember that these are normal sensations.
2. Soften into the chair and let your body relax, from your forehead to your neck, your shoulders, both arms, your abdomen, your hips, both thighs, both calves, and your ankles, to the tips of each toe.
3. While it may be daunting to recall the thoughts that are creating anger and resentment, it is important to identify them.
4. Use your breath to keep you grounded so that you do not get on the rollercoaster of your thoughts. Use each inhale and exhale to let go of those thoughts and feelings instead.
5. Use mindfulness meditation to observe the anger, guiding it towards patience and understanding while decreasing the force of its hold on you in the process.
6. Continue the process of exhaling anger and inhaling tranquillity. With each breath, you feel a sense of peace and calmness.
7. Remind yourself that anger is a natural reaction. However, if it is not managed appropriately it will

influence the decisions you make and how you feel, not from a positive place but from a place of negativity.

8. Now slowly begin to wiggle your fingers and your toes, gently opening your eyes and coming back to the room.

Noticing

There are times throughout your day when you experience a strong emotion, or perhaps several emotions. Usually, you do not actually notice that you're in such a state as it has become your usual default mode, part of your personality. Or so the mind will have you believe. Throughout this five-week journey, these states of emotions will become more apparent as you continue to practise awareness. This meditation can be used at any time of the day.

1. Begin by dropping an awareness into your body. Pay attention to any particular points where you feel an emotion. It may be in the side of your temples, your forehead, your neck, the upper part of your body, your hips or lower back, or perhaps lower down in your feet and calves.

2. Recognize the presence of an emotional experience. Rather than trying to avoid it, notice it with a kind awareness. Explore that feeling with patience.

3. Now soften and release the area of tension and breathe into it. Notice the air released from your lungs as you breathe out this feeling. Notice the abdomen moving inward and then outward, helping you to relax.

4. Repeat this in any other areas you feel are giving you discomfort. You do not need to label those feelings

or analyse them. Just be aware that a different feeling exists in one part of the body compared to another.

5. Use the breath to help nourish and heal you. Time does not exist at this moment, so for once there is no need to rush.

6. Now that you have given your body the attention it deserves, place your awareness at the top of your body – the mind.

7. Picture your mind as a vast ocean whose surface presents as deep crashing waves. You can notice the foam of the ocean and hear its fierce sounds.

8. However, deep beneath the surface there is a calmness and clarity. Too often you are caught up on top of the ocean, rarely going below it.

9. In this moment, you will allow yourself to go to that deep place, without fear. From this part of the ocean, place your gaze upwards and use your breath to stabilize you while you appreciate the depth and stillness of the ocean.

10. And as easily as that, the ocean that appeared vast and chaotic suddenly seems calm and clear. The waves of your mind start to settle. From this place, there is a serenity and peace you have not experienced in a while.

11. Take a deep breath in and absorb the moment. Let your thoughts and emotions settle, and gently flow along with the natural ebb and flow of the waves. Notice you are noticing.

Informal Mindfulness Practice

Reflect on This Week

Recall a practice or skill that you did this week. Then ask yourself the following questions and write down the answers:

- ◇ What went well?
- ◇ How did it make you feel?
- ◇ Did you notice any changes in your life, however small?
- ◇ What could you have improved on?

Mindful Walking

Suggested time: ten minutes daily.
This can be an indoor or outdoor activity.

1. Begin with an intention to be present while you walk.
2. Place your attention on your body, starting with the feet. Feel the connection with the ground, notice the position of your hips to stabilize your body and the position of your arms as you begin to move.
3. You are not forcing anything here, just paying attention to what your body wishes to do.
4. Notice how your body moves with each step.
5. How does your breathing alter during the walk?
6. Engage your senses to stay fully present, noticing the colours, the sounds, the smells, the weather against your face or the warmness of the room.
7. End the practice with gratitude, imagine your life without walking.

END OF WEEK THREE

By the end of this week, you will have begun to gain mastery of your inner voice. Adopting a growth mindset and reframing the inner dialogue that has stayed with you all these years will significantly improve the quality of your life.

WEEK FOUR:

PATHWAY TO 360-DEGREE SELF-HEALING

Mindfulness is not just a phase. It is a lifelong practice. To ensure your CAMPS stay erect, you must learn how to incorporate mindfulness in all aspects of your life.

Any self-healing programme must incorporate this kind of holistic approach. This week, you will learn how to use mindfulness principles on a daily basis and to stop surviving and start living.

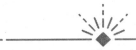

Here are some skills that you will learn
to cultivate this week:

**Embracing the modern world to
supplement your wellbeing**

**Incorporating mindfulness in
your personal sphere, such as in
your work and relationships**

**Using mindfulness alongside
other methods**

**Boosting your learning process
and adopting new skills**

The Digital Age

Regardless of our feelings about the digital age and its impact on society and individuals, it is here and an integral part of life. I feel it's important to discuss this, because phones, iPads, laptops and streaming services have become everyday necessities for most of us. Indeed, the internet is now viewed as a life essential in the same way as electricity, gas and water are.

Mindfulness is rooted in an ancient practice but this doesn't mean it cannot be embraced in the modern world. Various strategies can be used by the modern person to complement mindfulness. Studies have shown that between 40 and 80 per cent of the information doctors tell their patients is forgotten. To reinforce anything discussed during the consultation, I often reference articles on the internet and signpost patients to doctors on social media, some of whom have done wonderful work in engaging people with positive healthcare messages.

Mindfulness can be taught digitally in a variety of ways. There are specialist apps offering guided meditations and mindfulness exercises, as well as formal online mindfulness courses. Likewise, apps like TikTok, YouTube and Instagram all offer mindfulness resources to boost your daily practice. However, I would use these as additional resources rather than as your only resource. To gain the most out of mindfulness, we should practise it in an evidence-based way – that is, by undertaking a formal mindfulness programme.

Ten minutes of daily practice using an app is not going to give you lasting changes. A wellbeing programme must be educational and involve effort on your part. That effort should be made every day, to undo the negative thought patterns you have developed over the years and replace them with healthier ones.

Digital Toxicity

When talking about the digital age we also need to be mindful of digital toxicity. This has become prevalent among children as young as five right through to fully grown adults. Part of combatting digital toxicity is recognizing how addictive our devices are. They impede relationships at work and at home; and if used for long periods they inhibit not only personal growth but physical health too, due to prolonged immobility through their use. As my trainer Malath Shakir reminds me, in terms of disease impact, 'Sitting is the new smoking'. Symptoms of digital toxicity can include stress, sleep problems, addiction, depression and anxiety as well as feeling overwhelmed and frustrated.

Living mindfully means identifying and addressing the factors that stop you from staying in the present moment. For many of us that will involve turning off, setting boundaries and disconnecting from our devices. That is not to say we should discard them; but rather that we should use them more healthily, being mindful of how much technology is in our lives.

The latest research shows that people in the UK are spending over twenty-four hours every week online. Media company Ofcom conducted research in which many of the UK's 50 million internet users stated that the internet had a negative impact on them. Reported impacts included neglecting duties at work and home, being late, choosing holiday destinations based on the availability of internet access, and feeling tired because of sleep disruption caused by the internet. There is an opinion that it is mainly the youth who experience internet addiction and digital toxicity. However, research shows that many over the age of sixty-five also admit to having problems.

The problems of spending much of your time online can include low self-esteem, depression, anxiety, weight gain, lower emotional intelligence, social isolation, lack of exercise, loss of sense of time, low motivation and heightened attention-deficit symptoms. Your devices can suck the energy and life out of you; they take up your time – hours and hours of it – regardless of whether that's your intention. Some of you might use it as a distraction from how you are feeling, or as a means of escape. Again, this may be useful in short bursts but does not represent a positive life-changing approach to your problems.

Addicted to Our Devices

Experts have said that smartphones are as addictive as drugs such as cocaine because a similar release of dopamine occurs during use. Dopamine is a chemical that plays a role in motivation; for example, after exercise or eating something desirable, we get a release of dopamine that makes us feel good and motivates us to repeat that behaviour.

The brain has four dopamine pathways; three of these are considered 'reward' pathways and in cases of addiction, they are dysfunctional. When we're thinking about or experiencing a rewarding event, all three pathways are activated. A feel-good reward sequence follows. These associations become stronger and stronger every time they are activated. For example, the dopamine released during a positive, engaging conversation reinforces whatever led to that interaction. Likewise, positive online interactions such as receiving a like on a social-media post or a notification also results in dopamine release, and you'll seek to repeat that experience to get the same dopamine fix.

Social media apps understand this pathway very well and utilize it to keep you engaged as much as possible. Indeed, many of us when we're bored automatically find ourselves checking our phones out of pure habit rather than need. Many people report that if they misplace their phone they enter a mild panic state, which shows how the phone has become like an extra limb, an integral part of us.

When something starts to consume a lot of your time and your thoughts, interfering with daily functioning or spilling over into your work or personal life, this is the time to re-evaluate whether there is an addiction present. Digital and social-media detoxes are now available forms of therapy. In their 2023 study looking at the impact of body-positive social-media content on Italian women's mood and body image, Giulia Fioravanti and colleagues found that women who stopped using Instagram had greater life satisfaction. Those undergoing digital detox programmes often report improved mood and sleep.

Benefits of a Digital Detox

◇ Feeling of calm.

◇ Decreased stress.

◇ Increased productivity.

◇ Improved self-esteem.

◇ Decreased spending.

◇ Overcoming the feeling of missing out.

◇ Decreased body ache – a hunched posture can cause back and neck ache.

◇ Improved sleep – better release of melatonin helps you relax and enter the sleep state, which is inhibited by the glare of a screen.

If you think your technological use is unhealthy, you can limit it yourself using principles of mindfulness. Following the same process as you did for your life inventory, identify the stressors in your life. This time, make a note of all the different apps that you use and identify how much time you spend on each. You can do this over one week, in the form of a diary.

It's also worth noting which apps make you feel anxious and stressed and which ones bring you pleasure. In addition, keep a record of *why* you need to look at your phone. Is it because of boredom, or avoidance – putting off something unpleasant, such as a project or housework? Avoiding certain tasks for daily functioning will ultimately lead to unproductivity and feelings of low self-worth. Spending time on your device is not a healthy way to approach this.

There is an app for most things these days. For instance, you can use apps to track what you're using your phone for, to block social-media sites at certain times and to give you day-by-day comparative analysis of time spent on your phone.

Doctor's Prescription:
Mindful Digital Detox

Dissociate

Set an alarm or reminder and take time to disconnect from your device. I would physically remove the device by putting it away in another room rather than just setting it to silent, as the temptation to reach for it will be too much. Start with ten minutes' disconnection, and gradually work your way up.

Observe

Take note of your feelings and thoughts as you do this. Do you feel agitated or tense? Where do you feel this? Your jaw, your shoulders, in your abdomen? This is a great way to get to know your responses to stressful situations. Once you're familiar with how you react, you'll begin to observe these feelings much quicker and get a hold of them before they escalate.

Breathe

Once you've identified a feeling of anxiety or discomfort, start to replace it with some deep-breathing exercises, slowing down the stress response. Extend this to a formal mindfulness meditation practice for further relaxation.

Be Present

Be present in a situation instead of being present with your phone. This could mean engaging in meaningful conversations over dinner or listening to someone with full awareness. This will strengthen the relationships in your life. In time, you'll learn to master those external factors, taking control of your life and developing a strong internal focus from which you can draw strength.

Mindfulness at Work

Neuroscientists have demonstrated the benefits of mindfulness on the brain and how it can enhance cognitive function, including improved focus, concentration, problem-solving and decision-making. In addition, it can help reduce stress and anxiety, improve sleep and help build resilience. Mindfulness has been shown to reduce blood pressure and heart rates in individuals who practise it regularly.

Given its array of proven benefits on physical and psychological health, mindfulness practice should be integrated into the workplace. Every company should offer a mindfulness or wellbeing programme as standard, just like they do an induction and tour of the premises. Increasingly, mindfulness retreats are being organised as part of company team-building away-days. This is a promising start, but mindfulness should be incorporated into daily routine in much the same way as lunch breaks. Even a quick five-minute practice can centre us and improve how we perform.

Scheduling mindfulness or self-care breaks would do wonders in the workplace, improving mood and work performance.

In their 2015 study of mindfulness at work, Peter Malinowski and Hui Jia Lim concluded that 'mindfulness exerts its positive effect on work engagement by increasing positive affect, hope, and optimism, which on their own and in combination enhance work engagement ... Wellbeing, on the other hand, is directly influenced by mindfulness, which exerts additional indirect influence via positive affect, hope and optimism.'

In 2021, the Wellcome Institute produced a report regarding workplace mental health and recommended that all staff should be given access to mindfulness courses. This really shows how far mindfulness has come. The National Institute of Clinical Excellence, which many doctors refer to for guidance on treatment and diagnosis, stated in its 2022 report that mindfulness should be offered to 'all employees ... on an ongoing basis.' From Google and HSBC to Ford, LinkedIn and Apple, many big corporations already famously use mindfulness programmes for their employees. Fields such as education and mentoring can also benefit from mindfulness.

Getting Started

Our understanding of the workplace is no longer confined to offices or factories; nor are workers necessarily people who wear suits or uniforms. A stay-at-home parent is at work; catching up with projects or homework is being at work. A workplace is a location where you perform tasks and jobs, and this can vary widely. I think this chapter can apply to almost anyone.

Every person in your workplace or company can benefit from mindfulness, as outlined above. This can be from those in leadership positions to management to those who help keep your workplace in order, such as porters, cleaners, receptionists and other integral parts of your team. If your workplace is in the home, your spouse and your children are part of that space. The key concept to implement mindfulness in the workplace, wherever that may be, is consistency and accessibility. If something feels like too much effort and work, then your body's internal stress response will soon overwhelm you and convince you that this is something to abandon. The practice should be easily incorporated within your current way of life.

Incorporating mindfulness can be done in two ways: as a formal practice or an informal practice. You could set aside a specific time and place in your day to do a mindfulness meditation. If you've already started your day this way, remember there's no maximum amount of time you should allocate to meditation; you can recharge with another one! Informal mindfulness is the foundation to build your formal practice from. Informal mindfulness is conducted in everyday tasks, so you can do it as you go about your daily routine and gain the same benefits as you do from a formal mindfulness meditation practice.

Choose a Time and Place

The first step is to find a time of day when it will be easiest to implement your formal practice. If your mornings are too hectic or full of back-back meetings, then this won't be the best time. Your brain will be so caught up in the doing mode it's unlikely it'll be able to relax into the being mode. You may find that mid-afternoon has a slower pace and fewer demands; or perhaps the beginning of your lunchtime break will work for you. Your mind will also try its best to convince you that a meaningful break means having a snack or a cup of tea, catching up on social media, smoking a quick cigarette or making a phone call. However, a meaningful mindfulness meditation practice will have far more benefits than any of those activities if you wish to truly nourish your inner being and increase your productivity for the rest of the day. As little as ten minutes can bring you back to calmness and relaxation. People often become addicted to the benefits of mindfulness and soon want to practice more frequently.

Once you've identified a time of day, remember not to be too rigid about it – no two days are the same, so allow some flexibility. Unexpected events can happen and when they do you'll need to incorporate the practice at another time. Work may occasionally be so busy that it just doesn't happen at all; if that's the case, don't berate yourself and fall for the all-or-nothing principle, where you abandon the idea of practising mindfulness at work altogether.

Watch Your Inner Voice

The other 'tactic' your mind will use is the thought of your colleagues' reaction to you doing a meditation. Stereotypes about meditators still exist; usually it's assumed that it's females who meditate. However, attitudes in society are changing, and setting an example with confidence and leadership will work in your favour. Your wellbeing journey is not based on the opinion of others. Other people should not be the foundation upon which you make your decisions. Focus on the benefits that meditation will bring to your life, remain consistent and resolute, and soon your colleagues will come to know this is a part of you. In fact, they may even come to you to explore meditation further when they're facing their own difficulties. If the scrutiny of others becomes an issue that you find difficult to overcome, you may want to start with informal mindfulness practices or find a quiet space to practice a formal meditation where you will be alone and undisturbed. The hope is that wellbeing and meditation will soon become everyday language and an everyday practice, as normal as a coffee break.

Supplementing Your Practice

Journalling can be a useful tool when you're feeling particularly overworked and overwhelmed. You may wish to keep a separate 'work' journal, as the challenges in the workplace can be different to others in your life. A gratitude journal can provide a quick feel-good boost of dopamine.

Digitally Detox

Dampen down your sympathetic nervous system by setting aside specific times of the day to disconnect from emails and social media. Otherwise, this will activate your mind and you'll start to think about jobs that need doing, predicting outcomes, planning ... all of which take you away from being in the present moment.

Review

Identify what factors stopped you from practising mindfulness. Was it a matter of simply forgetting? Or perhaps time? Try to set alerts on your phone to give you a reminder. Scan your notes from the previous day and identify any quiet periods that could be used for meditation in the future. Ensure any journals you're using are in your work bag. Tell colleagues in advance what you're planning to do so that in your own mind this aspect of your programme doesn't snowball, giving power to unnecessary intrusive thoughts that hinder your wellbeing journey.

Mindful Leaders

Every job interview, regardless of the field, will always contain a question about leadership. This is a vital aspect of the workplace. Every individual must have leadership qualities, regardless of what position they have in the company. Leadership can involve anything from making simple decisions for yourself through to managing a whole team. Mindfulness can help significantly with the development of leadership qualities, through building self-awareness by understanding your blocks and fears, and by not avoiding those fears but instead working towards overcoming them with a kind curiosity and without self-criticism or feelings of worthlessness. Mindfulness also allows more focus and clarity in decision-making.

For those in leadership positions, empathy and compassion are strengths. They allow leaders to have better connections with their team members and to foster a supportive, open environment, encouraging better communication and a culture of innovation rather than inhibition. No doubt leadership roles are stressful, with their additional responsibilities; but mindfulness is also an effective stress-management tool.

For the workplace to function effectively, even leaders must be team players. Mindfulness has a role here through improved communication: it encourages us to be present, so we can show that we're fully engaged and respectful of our colleagues. Mindfulness encourages us to think about our role in the wider community and not just the self. This wider, collaborative approach leads to team cohesion. The principle of meta-awareness, which is the ability to observe experiences from an individual and the wider team perspective, goes very well with the principles of mindfulness. This allows you to foresee problems rather than simply waiting for them to happen.

In their 2018 study looking at the concept of team mindfulness, Lingtao Yu and Mary Zellmer-Bruhn found that when team members use mindfulness, conflicts are decreased and the teams remain more focused on their allocated activity, harnessing the different strengths within the group to achieve a common goal.

Doctor's Prescription:
Single-Tasking

It has long been thought that multitasking increases efficiency, but the reality is it dilutes the quality of performance. With your mind distracted by different tasks, mind wandering will affect your focus and concentration. Single-tasking improves not only the efficiency but also the quality of the work. Mindfulness allows you to be present in the moment, increasing awareness and attention. Mind wandering is extremely addictive and many of us unintentionally engage in it in most of, if not all areas of our lives.

When faced with a to-do list, try to tackle one thing at a time and notice how you don't feel so overwhelmed.

How to single-task:

○ Identify the task you wish to work on.

○ Allocate a specific time for this.

○ Minimize distractions to allow yourself to incorporate a learning state and get creative. This will help your focus.

○ Stay present, ensuring you give your full attention to the task in hand.

○ Watch out for signs of frustration – these might be physical, such as a clenched jaw or a feeling in your abdomen. Recognize this as possible stress. Take some time out and incorporate a simple meditation practice (any in the book that resonate with you). Then pick up where you left off.

Mindfulness in Daily Interactions

Your relationships with yourself and others can hugely impact the way that you feel. A toxic, negative relationship can take its toll mentally and physically, whereas a supportive, loving relationship can foster personal growth and wellbeing. We all seek to have positive relationships in our lives.

Mindfulness can have a role in this area. The practice of being fully present helps to acknowledge your emotions and thoughts relating to a situation or person. This creates empathy and compassion, which provides a platform for healthier communication. Mindfulness brings a fresh perspective to help build bonds of mutual respect, so you can cease to enter relationships as the victor or the victim.

Throughout their university years, medical students training to be doctors receive a great deal of teaching on effective communication, so that they can build relationships with their patients. After all, patients spend limited time with their doctor but must be comfortable opening up to them and trust them enough to follow any medical recommendations.

Building communication skills in your relationships will strengthen them and ultimately you will benefit from this bond. Below are three main key communication skills I use in my own consultations, which you can apply within the workplace or with friends and family in daily interactions.

1. Active listening. This involves being fully present during the conversation, without interruptions. I give my full attention by minimizing distractions such as my phone. I maintain eye contact and use supportive body language such as nodding to show that I am taking in what is being said – that the patient's words matter.

2. Empathy. Unlike sympathy, which is just a feeling, empathy is a powerful tool to understand what the patient is going through. Empathy can be demonstrated in several ways. For example, it can be expressed verbally, by using language such as, 'That must be difficult,' or by summarizing what the patient has said so that I truly understand their feelings and situation.

3. Use of open questions. Rather than asking the patient 'yes' or 'no' questions, I like to hear their narratives in their own words and give them space to tell me fully what is on their mind.

Rushing the patient also affects the rapport. Inevitably this means running late for the next patient sometimes, but I think that's a trade-off that everyone appreciates. Numerous studies have shown that a doctor's use of effective communication skills has a positive outcome on patient care, reducing their emotional distress, boosting their symptom control and leading to improvements in areas such as blood pressure and pain. As a doctor interacting with people daily, I cannot overemphasize how important communication is in relationships.

Dealing Well with Conflict

Having awareness and acceptance of your own and other people's emotions will help you develop listening skills as well as the ability to express your own thoughts. There will be ups and downs in any relationship, but good communication is key to dealing with situations of conflict. Communication allows you to explain where you're coming from and to develop teamwork skills so that you're open to learning and working together. I often see relationships being sabotaged when one person starts trying to mind-read what the other is thinking – those negative thoughts snowball quite quickly. This can lead to misunderstanding, which in turn leads to further anger and resentment. Mindfulness does not fit in with using the silent treatment, or jumping to conclusions or judgements, or focusing on the past as a strategy to deal with problems. Instead, allow space and time without interruption, where you are both fully present and accepting of each other.

In addition, practising gratitude and appreciation for those in your life is a very powerful way of dealing with negative thoughts regarding your partner or family. Gratitude doesn't have to be about grand gestures; you can appreciate people doing small things, such as not interrupting you when you were busy, making you a cup of tea, putting the laundry on, buying milk and paying bills, and for showing you qualities such as kindness, support, openness or freedom. You may think that these are all rights – they should be doing this anyway, so why should you be grateful? That is also true, but notice after practising gratitude how your feelings towards them change. Such a simple exercise benefits both you and your relationship.

Acknowledging Anger

Inevitably, doctors sometimes come across understandably angry patients. They may become angry after waiting too long to be seen while they are poorly, or because of delays in seeing a specialist, or after receiving devastating news such as a cancer diagnosis. The first step in dealing with these situations is to identify the patient's (or their relative's) feelings. This involves acknowledging not only what they are saying verbally, but also their body language, which can vary from aggressive posturing to being still and avoiding eye contact.

Once their feelings have been recognized, we then adjust our communication style to diffuse the situation. This can include keeping a calm tone of voice, remaining composed while speaking and adjusting our posture so that we're not crossing our arms and legs and appearing defensive. Patients, just like you and your loved ones, often just want to be heard. So, I always say to them that I can see they are upset; this offer of empathy is extremely valuable. At that moment, I'll try to put myself in their shoes, to understand why they're feeling the way they are, and encourage them to tell me more. I do this with active listening skills, such as nodding and eye contact, and by allowing them the space and freedom to communicate. Empathy makes the person feel that they are being listened to and that you care. Often that is all that is needed to diffuse a situation.

When you're faced with such a situation, the worst thing you can do is mirror the anger and raise your own voice. So, how about the other person? If you're coming from a positive place, displaying positive qualities and making an effort regarding your mindset, then the other person has no choice but to follow suit. It would be very difficult for them to continue to be in a state of negativity. However, please note that this advice does *not* apply if you're in a situation where you feel unsafe or threatened.

Communicating Well

This involves the same core principles of being present, being aware and non-judgement. In all relationships, communication is key. My own journey in this area continues to be up and down, but over time the downs occur less often and are a lot less deep.

For those in a caring role involving children, communication can be more challenging. Children often cannot verbalize how they're feeling, especially if they're young; but the same principle of acknowledgement is the first crucial step. Labelling feelings and thoughts is not always needed. It may be anxiety, maybe sadness or boredom; it could be a combination of everything. Reflecting on my parenting, when I bring judgement or I'm rushing to get somewhere on time, my sympathetic nervous system goes into overdrive. I think less clearly and I'm less patient. But through mindfulness, I have come to realize this. I can recognize the signs earlier on and utilize quick and simple mindfulness techniques to stop situations escalating and becoming worse.

Each stage of parenting brings its challenges and there are no doubt certain situations that act as triggers. For example, teenagers often express a high degree of self-interest; this combined with parental expectations can lead to disagreements. Meditation cultivates calmness and flexibility, which have a tremendously positive effect on decreasing parental stress.

In a similar way, in an effective doctor–patient relationship, the doctor should not just tell the patient what to do and expect them to follow. There should be a shared management plan to consider the patient's preferences and needs. As children get older, the parent-orientated approach cannot be used in the same way; asserting dominance goes against open communication and acknowledging the young person's needs.

Larissa Duncan, an associate professor of human development and family studies at the University of Wisconsin-Madison, describes a model of mindful parenting that encompasses five dimensions to the parent–child relationship:

◇ Listening with full attention.
◇ Non-judgemental acceptance of self and child.
◇ Emotional awareness of self and child.
◇ Self-regulation in the parenting relationship.
◇ Compassion for self and child.

Caring and leadership are symbiotic. We are all leaders in our own domains, making autonomous decisions about our lives, our household, our family and friends. Your leadership may be in a more formal capacity within a company or group of people. It may be permanent or fleeting. The qualities of a successful leader are being supportive, communicating clearly, commitment, openness to differing approaches and the ability to reflect upon things that went well and not so well. By paying attention and being present, all these factors can be greatly enhanced. Paying attention to your interactions with others, recognizing their feelings with empathy and being aware of your own limitations can all help to avoid stressful situations and create a harmonious environment.

Dealing with Loss

There are times in all our lives when we experience loss or disappointment. This could be the loss of a loved one or a relationship, or maybe the loss of part of yourself through a profound event. Loss could be something that you missed out on – perhaps a job or a role. You may have lost something tangible that was very precious to you. Loss is very personal. In fact, many people who have experienced the loss of someone, or something, feel that others cannot provide empathy as they cannot possibly understand how they feel.

Loss can be a mixture of emotions and difficult to define; perhaps it is an overwhelming feeling of sadness, or pain or grief. Loss can induce fear, because it may involve change. As with any challenging situation, the first step is to acknowledge these feelings without judgement.

This is the beauty of mindfulness; it creates a safe space to process our experiences without feeling belittled or that our distress is being minimized.

Doctor's Prescription:
Developing Empathy

There will be challenging times in any relationship, where patience and understanding momentarily leave your thought pattern and can be replaced with feelings of anger, betrayal and hurt. Have these negative thoughts ever benefitted you? Are you able to think clearly in this emotional state? Next time you are feeling this way, I would like you to be honest with yourself about these questions.

Let's try something new. I would like you to cultivate empathy in a difficult interaction. Empathy is a tool that enables us to reduce stress in both ourselves and the person we're interacting with.

Here are five steps to developing empathy:

○ **Minimize distractions.** Show the other person that they matter. Put away your phone and do not try to multitask while you're having the conversation.

○ **Minimize the need to talk.** For this moment, let them get their words out. Once they have finished, without interruptions, relay your thoughts. You may feel a tendency to finish their sentences or jump in with your analysis. Hold off.

- ○ **Show that you are listening.** Do this using verbal and non-verbal cues. A simple, 'I understand,' can provide great comfort, as can an open posture – whereas crossing your arms and legs can appear defensive.

- ○ **Withhold judgement.** Often people want the space to be heard, rather than to be offered advice. Clarify what they are looking for so you can facilitate the interaction. Advice often comes with judgement, which can include judgement of the person that has come to you.

- ○ **Be present to their feelings, and your own.** If they are getting agitated or angry, be careful to not get caught up in those emotions too. Mirroring their behaviour and ending up with both of you experiencing heightened emotions can cloud your decision-making skills and add to the tension rather than diffusing conflict.

Mindful Learning

Mindfulness is a powerful tool for any person involved in learning. While we often think of learning as a student in school, college or university, we are all learning at various stages of our lives – whether that's in a new job or trying to work a new gadget or master a new skill. You will be familiar by now with how mindfulness can benefit your life. It is particularly relevant to learning because it can improve your focus, memory and ability to retain information. Staying in the present moment and reducing mind wandering allows us to fully engage with whatever it is that we're learning. This is needed now more than ever before, as the endless distractions of the modern world can significantly impact on our attention and ability to focus.

There are different schools of thought regarding mindfulness and its impact on achievement, but several sources confirm a positive association. In their 2019 study looking at mindfulness and academic achievement, Camila Caballero and colleagues found that grade-point averages and standardized test scores for maths and literacy were improved with mindfulness programmes. In addition to their improved performance, students across all demographics had better attendance records and fewer suspensions.

In 2011, Britta K. Hölzel and colleagues used MRI scans to look at the effects of mindfulness practice on the brain, and confirmed that there were structural differences in the brains of those who meditate. There was an increase in grey matter in the hippocampus (a part of the brain involved learning and memory) as well as a decrease in grey matter in the amygdala (a part of the brain that plays a role in anxiety and stress).

Mindfulness is now being introduced in many educational and workplace settings, but it is a subject in its own right – and like any other subject it requires 'homework'. It is dose-dependent: the more time you invest in it, the greater the results. According to Public Health England, depression has been attributed to 109 million lost working days annually in England and 61 per cent of adults with mental-health conditions do not access treatment. There continues to be a backlog to access NHS mental-health services, exacerbated by Covid. As a doctor, I see the effects of poor mental health and we need to put as much emphasis on prevention as we do on treatment.

Giving people the tools to cope with mental-health problems that they can access for the rest of their lives will hugely benefit the NHS and our society as a whole. Rather than 'introducing' mindfulness, it should be conducted in the way that is supported by the most research, which is an eight-week course delivered by an experienced practitioner. Mindfulness not only benefits the individual student but also the wider community.

Doctor's Prescription:
Mindful Learning Top Tips

○ Repeat affirmations that align with success in your chosen area of learning.

○ Visualize the steps needed, such as effective revision for a test/new job, as well as imagining yourself doing well.

○ Check-in with yourself. Notice if you're feeling particularly anxious and incorporate some mindful breathing techniques. Feet on floor, body on chair (FOFBOC) is a common practice where you take a few moments to just stop and be in the present moment.

○ Breathe deeply while you focus on your task, which will stimulate the parasympathetic nervous system and allow you to enter the relaxation state. As you breathe out, your blood pressure and heart rate will start to lower, and you will begin to feel relaxed. The 7/11 breathing exercise is very effective: here, you breathe in for a count of seven and breathe out for a count of eleven. The beauty of this is that the results are quite quick. Like most mindfulness practices, it can be done at any time, in any place, and needs no other physical resources.

Supplemented Practices

As a healthcare professional, I have an open mind regarding all the practices outlined below; I believe they represent a step towards holistic medicine, which every doctor advocates. These therapies show promising evidence and can enhance wellbeing by relieving stress and improving the overall quality of life. As a fundamental pillar of medical ethics, patients should have autonomy in their choices. I can help in this process by encouraging patients to actively invest in their self-care, in whatever way works for them providing it is not harmful to their health and is backed by scientific evidence. However, I would not suggest that the following therapies are used to *replace* conventional medical treatment, as patient safety is always the utmost priority.

Aromatherapy

The word *aroma* means fragrance or smell. Aromatherapy, like many practices, is now enjoying a resurgence, although it has been around for centuries, especially in the Far East. It involves the use of concentrated plant-based essential oils. Aromatherapy is often used in a wide range of conditions, from migraines to the common cold to pain relief, and offers an overall sense of calmness.

Essential oils are extracted from parts of different plants, such as the flowers or leaves, using pressure such as steam. The oils are made up of a mixture of various elements, including hydrocarbons, alcohol, phenols and terpenes. In undiluted form, they can be potent for work on pressure points. It is thought that the stimulation properties of these oils are significant because their structure resembles actual hormones.

When the oils are inhaled, the particles travel from your nose to the brain via the olfactory nerve. The brain picks up the signal and the amygdala – the stress centre of the brain – is activated. This causes the release of neurotransmitters such as serotonin and endorphins, which help to produce a calming effect on the mind and body. This is the basis on which aromatherapy works.

French chemical engineer René-Maurice Gattefossé pioneered the use of modern-day essential oils. Due to his natural interest in raw materials, he met with farmers in France who grew lavender. As a chemist, he was often involved in experimenting. Unfortunately, an explosion in one of his laboratories resulted in severe burns – and it was this incident that led him to conduct his groundbreaking research into essential oils. He put his burned hands in the nearest container he could find, which happened to hold lavender oil. He was astonished at how quickly his burns healed. During the First World War, he used essential oils to heal wounded soldiers, using lemon and clove for their antiseptic properties. This is how he became known as the 'father of aromatherapy'.

Common essential oils:

- ⋄ Lavender – promotes sleep and relieves anxiety
- ⋄ Eucalyptus – for nasal decongestion (Vicks decongestant contains eucalyptus)
- ⋄ Tea tree – antibacterial
- ⋄ Peppermint – aids digestion
- ⋄ Ginger – anti-nausea
- ⋄ Chamomile – stress relief
- ⋄ Rosemary – focus

The appeal of aromatherapy is that it is natural and non-invasive, and has whole-body benefits. Advocates say that it is also involved in prevention and cure. It may be used on its own or as an adjunct to medication and other forms of therapy. However, there may be a lack of expertise and knowledge on how this could be done safely.

Research in helping medical symptoms looks promising, although more work is needed before we see this practice advocated by mainstream medical doctors. The field of aromatherapy is nonetheless an exciting area of research in wellbeing. For example, a 2004 study by Annarica Calcabrini and colleagues showed that tea tree oil and Terpinen-4-ol were able to halt the growth of cancer cells.

At present there is no regulatory body for essential oils,

so ingredients and their quantities may not always be clearly listed on the bottle. Although side effects are few, John Hopkins Medical Centre advocates use of the popular household essential-oil diffusers to be tailored to individual needs. For example, an essential oil for an adult may be therapeutic but could have adverse consequences for a baby. Similarly, the inhalation of vapours may be unsuitable for people with certain medical conditions. Essential oils applied to the body may also produce an allergic reaction. The message here therefore is to take caution, do your due diligence before using them and contact a medical professional if you feel unwell.

Vision Boards

The use of vision boards – also known as mood boards – is advocated by many self-health experts. You may have used them when designing a room, to visualize how the space will be. They can be literal boards or just pieces of paper, but they'll contain words and pictures, or just pictures, of any shape or size, whether cut from a magazine, printed from the internet or drawn by you.

Vision boards are used as a motivational tool, to set out your goals and represent what you want to achieve. They are a useful tool, as the brain can process images faster than it can process words. Once you achieve your chosen goals, your vision board can be updated. This itself is quite satisfying. Your goals can be small or large; there are no limits in how you use a vision board. However, just making a vision board doesn't mean your dreams will come true. To get the most out of it, you should also use the practice of visualization. When you look at your chosen images, imagine that you already have whatever it is that you're seeking, remembering that your brain cannot distinguish between what is real and imaginary. This exercise will be strengthened by repetition.

Visualizing the steps involved in achieving your goal will have a beneficial effect – so for example, if you wish to be a certain weight, you should visualize yourself eating the right foods or exercising. Vinoth K. Ranganathan and colleagues found in their 2004 study that people who did virtual workouts in their imagination increased their strength by 35 per cent, which demonstrated the mind's ability to exert influence over the body.

Neuroscientist Dr Tara Swart says that vision boards can 'prime the brain to grasp opportunities that may otherwise have gone unnoticed'. This process of 'value tagging' essentially means that the brain will identify the selected information as important and therefore will not discard it but instead imprint it onto your subconscious. Dr Swart recommends doing this just before you go to bed. I would suggest you also refer to it throughout the day, so that your mind accepts the vision as real.

Biochemically, it is thought that vision boards can help you achieve your goals through familiarization. When you first think of a new event, your brain goes into survival mode and the sympathetic nervous system is activated to release stress hormones. As you start to think about that event more and more, you become comfortable with it and consequently there's a dampening of that nervous pathway.

Within your brain, there is a group of neurons called the reticular activating system (RAS), which is involved in attention and arousal. When information is sent to that system, it determines which bits are the most important and then communicates with other parts of the brain, helping it to focus. It is thought that there's a connection between vision boards and the RAS, whereby focusing your attention on a specific goal activates the pathway that helps you to achieve it by directing your awareness to it.

If you have a physical vision board, I suggest placing it where you can view it several times a day, to strengthen the neural pathways. Vision boards can also be created on your phone via an app, and you could set a reminder to look at them several times a day. Be specific about what you want; and it's worth taking time to decide your goals for the next year. You could divide them into different areas of your life, such as work, money, health, travel and relationships, but the goals don't need to be physical entities. You could visualize spiritual growth, cultivating kindness, or having more patience. You may want to then draw up a list and prioritize what you want to accomplish first. It's important not to include too many things on your vision board, as you could become easily overwhelmed. When selecting your images, go for those that elicit a positive strong emotion.

You can arrange the pictures in any way you wish; they don't have to be neat or in order – they can be as messy as you like. There is no right or wrong way to do it, so just use whatever resonates with you. If you cannot find a graphical representation, you can simply put the words on your board. It is well known that 90 per cent of the information transmitted to your brain is in the visual form. The brain likes the visual in vision boards.

I would also advise keeping your vision board where only you can see it. I find that when people know their vision board will be seen by others they are not truly open and honest. For example, you may find that you limit your goals because you fear you'll be laughed at. There should be no limit to your goals, regardless of whether anyone else believes they are achievable or not. The voice in your head may also limit your ambitions so it's worth watching out for that inner critic: do not let it be a part of this process.

When I started using a vision board it was a big A3 piece of paper. I find it amazing that I only have a few pictures on there now, as one by one my goals have been achieved.

Doctor's Prescription:
Your Vision Board

A year ago, my vision board featured an image of a book. I did not know what the title was or what it was about, but I put my name on it in big font. I visualized myself as an author – and here I am. Because vision boards represent goals in your life, you can include whatever you wish, from travel and jobs to weight, relationships and skills.

Here are my five steps to creating a vision board:

○ Set your specific goals and go into detail. For example, if you're visualizing having a house, give details of the house number, its front door, driveway and number of bedrooms.

○ Stick to no more than five goals.

○ Convert your goals into visual-image form, using pictures from magazines or the internet and so on.

○ Now decide where you'll place your board and

when you'll look at it every day. Set a reminder for this practice.

○ Add some positive affirmations.

Sound Therapy

I came across sound therapy in my quest for wellbeing and self-care practices – I've tried most things and if something is without obvious side effects, I'm always willing to give it a go. Like many of these therapies that are undergoing a modern resurgence, sound therapy has been around for many years. The indigenous Australian population were well known to have used ancient didgeridoos for healing.

Sound therapy is another form of complementary medicine. It is well documented that music can prompt mental and physical responses. Think about what happens when your favourite song comes on while you're driving your car; or imagine attending a spa session, where you'd expect the music to be relaxing and instrumental rather than loud rock. Music is known to provoke the release of endorphins and dopamine as well as decreasing stress hormones such as cortisol.

A 2017 study by Tamara L. Goldsby and colleagues looked at Tibetan bowl meditation and its effect on mood and anxiety. The results showed that there was an improvement in these areas and that the feeling of spiritual wellbeing was increased in all participants. The author concluded that conditions such as heart disease, diabetes and mental health could benefit from this type of intervention, because all these conditions are linked to stress. If a practice can lower stress and anxiety, then activating the parasympathetic nervous system will help lower blood pressure and have an overall positive effect on the cardiovascular system.

Sound therapy works through the senses, like aromatherapy. It uses instruments such as crystal or Tibetan bowls, shakers, chimes, gongs tuning forks and drums. It can also involve the voice. Sound-therapy sessions offer an energizing treatment while deep relaxation is also achieved. Sessions are tailored to your condition or body part, and instruments are played in a specific order. The practice can be combined with yoga, and the process and outcome are similar to meditation. Binaural beats – where two tones of differing frequency are played simultaneously – are also now a popular method to reduce anxiety.

In a 2015 study, Lili Naghdi and colleagues looked at the effect of sound stimulation on the condition of fibromyalgia, a syndrome that causes widespread body pain, tiredness and low mood. Female participants attended two sessions over five weeks of sound therapy. Before and after each session, they were asked to fill in a questionnaire that included markers of sleep and pain as well as movement. No side effects were reported, and the volunteers reported significant clinical improvement in their symptoms. Sounds with slower melodies and lower frequencies were all thought to have the most relaxing effect. Sounds of nature, such as rain, also helped the nervous system.

How sound therapy works is still not fully understood. There is a hypothesis that sound therapy stimulates receptors in the body that then go on to block pain transmission. Further studies have also looked at the role of music in other painful conditions, such as arthritis, menstrual and back pain.

The advantage of this type of practice is that it is easily accessible, because you can simply download songs. And any type of self-healing that can benefit you is worth trying; you may find it extremely beneficial alongside your mindful way of living.

Acupuncture

The NHS website has a page dedicated to acupuncture, which it describes as a treatment derived from ancient medicine. The National Institute of Health and Care Excellence (NICE) recommends acupuncture for chronic pain, headache and migraines and prostatitis symptoms. Funding is available through some GP practices.

Acupuncture involves the insertion of needles through the skin at certain points on your body. Chinese medicine recognizes that we all have a flow of energy or life force (chi), and that in certain conditions these pathways (meridians) are disrupted. The insertion of needles is thought to restore the flow of energy. In modern medicine, it is thought that acupuncture points coincide with specific points in the nervous system, which when activated release chemicals such as endorphins – which in turn cause physical changes in the body that promote wellbeing.

At present there is no regulatory body for acupuncture in England, so the NHS advises patients to access treatment through a regulated health professional, such as a doctor or nurse. It is also advisable that symptoms are first diagnosed by a recognized medical-health professional. Acupuncture is not advised for people with bleeding disorders or who have an allergy to metals, or who are taking certain medications, such as anticoagulants. There are rare side effects, including infection, but generally the procedure is considered safe.

The National Centre for Complementary and Integrated Health found positive effects of acupuncture following analysis of data from twenty studies of those with painful conditions such as arthritis and headaches. For most participants, these benefits continued for a year after treatment.

A common treatment plan involves attending one to two sessions of acupuncture per week, for about six to eight weeks, depending on the number and severity of the conditions to be treated; but you should discuss this with your acupuncture practitioner. This can be a mindful activity itself or a practice alongside this five-week course for overall wellbeing and stress relief.

Meditations

Meditations for Week Four are designed to encourage personal growth by focusing on the camp itself. You will foster the feelings of being safe and abundance by working in harmony with your body's physiology.

The Camp

You have arrived at the most important part of your journey: your sanctuary. Your healing starts here.

1. Begin to relax by focusing on your breath, taking a full, deep breath in and exhaling out, watching your chest rise and fall with each breath.
2. Bring to mind the image of a camp: a place of shelter where you feel safe and warm. Visualize all the details of this camp – its colours, textures, shapes; the space

and the smells inside.

3. You may be able to hear the wind howling outside, or the rain pouring onto your tent; or perhaps it's a hot sunny day. The camp provides shelter from every element in your life.

4. How does it feel to be here? Notice your breathing and any sensations throughout your body. This is a place of relaxation.

5. Develop this feeling by remembering a time when you felt proud of something – an accomplishment, or a positive comment, or perhaps reaching a personal goal. Remember how you physically felt at that time. What emotions were going through your mind?

6. Really experience that feeling of excitement and now let that positivity radiate throughout your body while you sit in this safe place.

7. As you continue to remain here, bring up a feeling of gratitude. Feel grateful for all the other camps in your life that have helped you so far. Those camps are a representation of supportive relationships, from family to friends to colleagues. Other camps could be your house, your apartment, your clothes, the food and water that is so readily available. Be grateful for everything that supports you right now.

8. Through these exercises you will learn more about how you react, so where do you feel this emotion or gratitude? Sit with this feeling for a while.

9. Life is so busy with people and tasks demanding your time and attention. In this camp, just relax; there is no need to do anything at all.

10. This camp allows yourself to heal and it feels good to

be here, taking time from your day to intentionally nourish yourself.

Plenty in Abundance

Generating a feeling of abundance is a prerequisite for ensuring you have abundance in your life. Think of something good in your life – what comes to mind? Delve deeper, rather than just thinking of material abundance, such as having a house, money, or a job. Think of the good qualities that others appreciate you for, such as kindness, honesty, or being a team player. Often we take things for granted, but lessons are there in our everyday lives and usually it's noticing the small things that opens the way for abundance.

1. The most honourable lesson in your life is your breath. Take some deep, intentional breaths. Fully inhale, expanding your abdomen and chest, pause for three seconds and then exhale feeling a deep sense of relaxation. Repeat this another four times.
2. This is a simple practice, but now you have filled yourself with nourishing oxygen that is freely available and abundant to you. This conscious breathing is a quick and powerful tool to amplify the feeling of positivity.
3. If there is something in particular that you wish to have in abundance, bring it to mind in specific terms – for example, as a specific date or goal, or in a specific timeframe.
4. Make an intention to dedicate effort to your goal and visualize yourself doing so now. You are taking the necessary steps with ease and confidence.

5. Notice how that feels. Believe in your mind, in your heart and in your body that you have successfully accomplished your goal.

6. Lastly, have trust – trust in the process and in yourself so that you do not overthink or let those feelings of self-doubt and self-criticism creep in. If you notice they are, reframe the thoughts and visualize yourself reaching your goals effortlessly.

Inner Apartments

Your apartment is your place of security and safety. It does not have to be grand or lavish but is somewhere special that belongs only to you. In time, coming back to this inner apartment that you've created will be the most wonderful pastime you've developed for yourself.

1. Notice where you are right now, as you begin to settle yourself. Notice the energy in your body and your mind. Is your mind active with racing thoughts? Thoughts about the day ahead or the events of yesterday?

2. Have those thoughts affected your physical body? Notice any areas of tightness or tension. Begin to observe where in your body you feel this the most.

3. This state of being is not your inner sanctuary. Your safe place is a place of peace and calm. A natural state that you can return to at any time.

4. Think of your active mind as a shaken snow globe, thoughts all over the place and swirling in every direction. Chaotic. Agitated. Reduced visibility. You're unable to see or to think clearly.

5. Now just pause. Stay still with your breath. Move your attention from your mind to the breath. There is no need to force anything in this moment, just pay attention and breathe.

6. If you let the snow globe be, without any other action, the snow will settle itself. As the flakes return to the bottom, the picture becomes clearer.

7. Without any effort, peace is restored. By observing the physical sensation of the breath, your thoughts will begin to settle. Nothing else is needed.

8. Some snowflakes take longer than others to return to the bottom of the globe. That is no cause for concern. They will all eventually return home, to their starting position.

9. Some of your thoughts will want to linger in the same way; your mind will want to keep a hold of them. That is no cause for concern. Acknowledge the thoughts, return to the breath whenever this happens, and eventually those thoughts will no longer impact your return to a natural relaxation state.

10. Continue to relax in the waves of your breath, noticing the feeling of each exhalation and each inhalation. The physical body follows the mind; as the mind settles, so your physical body begins to relax. Notice those areas of tension. How do they feel now?

11. Without any extra effort, you have entered a state of deep relaxation. If any sounds around you occur while you are here, embrace them. They are part of your experience. If any interruptions occur, there's no need to get annoyed. Just let things be.

12. Return to the breath. Do you notice any sensations of

warmth or coolness? The breath may feel cool around your lips as you breathe, as the gases of carbon dioxide and oxygen exchange in a friendly encounter, passing each other in an instant, keeping you alive, without any effort. So much of your body is supporting you right now.

13. You may drift off into thought once more. Do not label having a thought as something negative. You do not need to clear your mind of thoughts; rather, you want to be in a state where they don't engulf you.

14. You want to be in a state where you're not getting lost in the storyline of thoughts. But the mind does not always want to settle so easily, so let it play for a brief moment. Acknowledge it, then watch your thoughts settle one by one.

15. Your inner apartment is the present moment. It may have been a while since you returned but now you are here. You came back. And now that you have found your way, you can return any time.

Serenity in Sleep

Sleep is a powerful place. Maintaining a good sleep pattern has been linked to a reduced risk of developing medical problems such as diabetes and heart disease. Poor-quality sleep negatively affects your concentration and mood the next day. Sleep deserves it very own meditation; it's only fitting that you use this meditation often, to contribute to your overall health.

1. Take time to find a comfortable position or posture in your bed, and adjust the pillow or duvet or any other accessories you need to feel relaxed.

2. You will now enter a phase of stillness and calm. Begin by taking a few breaths, breathing in consciously, not trying to change the breath in any way.

3. In order to pay attention to the breath, you may find it helpful to place one hand on top of the other, on your chest or upper abdomen. This allows you to connect to the breath and feel its movement in and out.

4. As you stay with your breath, notice the points of contact with the bed, such as the back of your head, your upper back, or your sides, your pelvis, the back of your legs, or the sides of your legs. Fully sink into the bed and let it take all your weight.

5. Here you feel protected and safe. You can let go of any demands of the day. There is no doing in this moment, just resting.

6. Thoughts may try to disturb this experience, but do not be angry at the mind. Instead, acknowledge those thoughts and let them drift away with ease.

7. With each breath, let go of any tension any tightness. Start with your face, your forehead; let it relax. Now the muscles around the eyes; soften them, unclench the jaw and relax the tongue.

8. Work your way down to the neck and the shoulders, letting them drop and sink into the mattress. Let your arms relax loosely wherever they feel comfortable, not forcing the body to be in any particular position. Now pay kind attention to your lower back and release any discomfort here by breathing into it.

9. Finally, focus your attention on your two legs, which carry you wherever you want to go throughout your day. Bring awareness to both feet; breathe into them,

for they have worked hard to carry the full weight of your body.

10. Let the whole body relax and continue to breathe as you slowly drift off, entering a realm of rejuvenation and repair.

Activate Your Biological Response

Remember, the breath is the key to relaxation. In this calm state, your mind is clear, allowing you to make choices necessary to improve your wellbeing, inside and out.

1. Adopt a position to undertake a meditation practice. Start to breathe slowly, in and out through your nose, with each exhale lasting as long as each inhale.

2. Deep breathing allows the activation of the parasympathetic nervous system, sending a signal to your brain that it is safe and providing it with much-needed oxygen.

3. With this part of the nervous system now promoted, your heart rate, breathing rate and blood pressure will start to lower. This is also known as the 'rest and digest' system.

4. Inhale for a count of four, hold your breath for a count of four, then exhale for a count of four. Repeat this process for up to ten breaths.

5. If you feel comfortable, deepen this practice by increasing to a count of six.

6. In this deep relaxation phase, your body can restore energy and promote digestion and aid recovery by increasing blood flow to major organs.

7. You spend most of your time activating the sympathetic nervous system but now you are maintaining an inner equilibrium, by promoting a state of calmness. Through the breath, this can be achieved very quickly and simply.

8. In this safe space, you break away from the daily demands and unconscious repetitive habits that hold you back from activating the parasympathetic nervous system.

9. Continue to stay here, knowing that you are fully capable of deeply relaxing; you need only to acknowledge this. Relaxation is your right and a natural state for you.

Informal Mindfulness Practice

Reflect on This Week

Recall a practice or skill that you did this week. Then ask yourself the following questions and write down the answers:

- ◇ What went well?
- ◇ How did it make you feel?
- ◇ Did you notice any changes in your life, however small?
- ◇ What could you have improved on?

Mindful Grounding

Suggested time: ten minutes daily.

This is also referred to as 'earthing'. It is a way to reconnect with nature and your place in the world. And to remind yourself of the Earth's ecosystem, which sustains and supports life on the planet.

1. Walk outdoors barefoot, in your garden or front yard.
2. Pay attention to the soles of your feet as they connect with the ground. This will allow you to reconnect to nature.
3. Stay in the present moment by being fully aware of your surroundings.
4. Breathe deeply, in and out, while you are here. You will feel a sense of freedom and relaxation.

END OF WEEK FOUR

By the end of Week Four, you will really begin to see the progress you have made as you have finally built your camp. You have made it. Everything in your life has been lessons so that you can arrive at this precise moment.

WEEK FIVE:

SCIENCE OF STRESS AND SELF-CARE

The future is bright. Understanding the science behind the concepts will make sure that your CAMPS remain firmly rooted and that the path ahead is illuminated, because you understand how it works in synergy with your natural being.

During Week Five you will discover your internal stress response and learn how to control it, enabling you to deal with daily stressors and giving you the tools for lifelong wellbeing.

Here are some skills that you will learn
to cultivate this week:

**Developing positive
pathways in the brain**

**Managing difficulties that
come your way**

Visualizing your goals

**Creating a mindful way of
life for the future**

The Science of Stress Management

In many cultures, the idea of the individual and the pursuit of happiness are of the utmost importance. This has led to great advances, especially in the technological world and the recreational activities that people devote much of their non-working time to. However, while society evolves and advances, our collective mental health is the worst that it has ever been. While the idea of wellbeing has gained popularity, achieving it remains elusive. The rate at which the volume of available wellbeing resources such as books, podcasts and social-media channels is growing signifies the void in people's lives.

As babies, our needs were very simple: to be fed, to be changed, to have enough sleep, to be in a comfortable temperature. Given available resources, these are relatively easy needs to meet. As we grow older, our needs became more complicated. We begin to have more complex emotional needs, such as companionship through conversation and bonding over similar interests, strengthening the feeling of being loved. Our social needs evolve from our desire to have a sense of belonging. Our intellectual needs grow too and we must learn new skills, from language to maths to problem-solving. Finally, many of us have the need for spiritual fulfilment, which religion or activities such as meditation help us to achieve.

Meeting all these demands is not easy. There's no guidebook to tell you how to be happy; it's not something that gets taught in schools, and there's no single course you can learn it from. It's not something that you can easily learn from others either – in fact, the people who care for you and raised you don't know the answer themselves, so how were they meant to pass on the right knowledge? Your caregivers or parents had their own challenges and stresses; they didn't know how to address their own needs, so they couldn't possibly know how to address yours.

The Stress Spiral

When all these various needs are unmet, there follows a downward path to unfulfillment and unhappiness. And without the knowledge of how to fulfil them, we turn to other sources of pleasure that may themselves be harmful – for example, excessive drinking, using recreational drugs, emotional eating, social-media or gaming addiction.

Stress then manifests as a variety of feelings and physical symptoms, which include everything from insomnia to forgetfulness and feeling sad, tired or disorganized, to having difficulties making decisions and feeling irritable, frustrated, overwhelmed and nervous. This becomes a vicious cycle where the 'remedies' we use are often also stressful; so these things compound each other, and magnify the overall effects.

Good Stress

However, not all stress is harmful. Acute stress is natural and helpful and it's through this design that humans were able to evolve. When we have exams, or a specific task to complete at work, are running for a bus, about to have a meeting, or even about to cook, our bodies must mentally and physically prepare. We don't even realize they're preparing; it all happens without any conscious doing on our part.

Once the decision to undertake a certain task is registered in the brain, hormones are released that activate our internal stress response. Stress in this case does not have the negative connotations we usually think of; it just means an imminent event registered by your brain. So, once this pathway is activated, we are ready for the task at hand, we can do it successfully and when it's done the body can relax. This is known as 'eustress'. When we meet these tasks successfully we feel good, and that motivates us to do more. Our personal skills grow as we develop confidence and resilience.

This internal phenomenon is known as the 'fight or flight' response. The amygdala in the brain, which processes emotions, sends a signal to another area in the brain, called the hypothalamus. The hypothalamus acts as a control centre and through the nervous system it will communicate the need for fight or flight to the entire body.

This activation causes the release of the hormone adrenaline, which in turn causes your heart rate to increase, your blood pressure to elevate and glucose to release into the bloodstream.

This prepares the body for what is about to occur. The glucose provides energy, the elevated heart rate allows quicker and greater blood flow to vital organs as blood vessels become dilated. Along with a quicker breathing rate, this aids oxygen availability. Your pupils also dilate, which increases your vision so you can make a visual assessment of your surroundings, and your hearing becomes sharper. This natural stress response – the sympathetic nervous system – has been present since the start of humankind.

Action > Reaction

The human body is remarkable. For every action, there is a reaction. The opposite of the fight-or-flight response is the relaxation response – the parasympathetic nervous system. The human body is a combination of intricate systems that together work in perfect balance. Dr Herbert Benson of Harvard Medical School was the first to talk about this relaxation pathway. When an event activated by the sympathetic nervous system is over, this too is acknowledged by the brain. It then switches off the sympathetic nervous system and switches on the parasympathetic nervous system, to counteract the effects of adrenaline.

Through the vagus nerve, it downregulates the body by releasing the hormone acetylcholine, which slows down our breathing and heart rate and lowers our blood pressure, so that the body returns to its natural, pre-event state where recovery can occur. The parasympathetic nervous system is otherwise known as the 'rest and digest' mode and is also responsible for your metabolism. This system is like a messenger to the brain, telling it what's happening, whereas the sympathetic nervous system gives the brain orders.

These two carefully orchestrated systems work in harmony

with each other as partners, and together make up the body's autonomic nervous system. Both systems are activated in an instant, without any conscious input, and have important roles in everyday life.

Stress Responses

Our ancestors utilized this phenomenon when they faced 'real' threats, such as being chased by predators. In prehistoric times, threats tended to be more physical than mental, while today, we're much less likely to find ourselves being chased by a lion while out hunting. Modern-day threats are increasingly mental, ranging from cyberbullying to harassment or toxic colleagues and family dynamics.

However, the brain cannot distinguish between physical and mental threats, or discern what's real or imagined; all will activate the sympathetic nervous system, releasing adrenaline. So, the same stress responses are activated whether we're in a traffic jam or running away from a lion. Even thinking about past stressful events will put us in fight-or-flight mode. This means that many of us have an internal chemical imbalance.

The sympathetic nervous system is switched on far more often than the parasympathetic nervous system is. This occurs because of our thoughts. A lot of our time and energy is spent dealing with stressful thoughts, mainly concerning the past and the future, with little regard for the present moment. It's this stress that is harmful: when the body is continuously in a stress response and cannot relax and return to its natural state. We call this *chronic* stress. It's that sense of being overwhelmed, low and under pressure for a prolonged period of time. Chronic stress commonly happens following a major life event, such as losing a job, bereavement, or moving house. It has more far-reaching implications and often there's no immediate solution.

Stress can have a detrimental impact on your immune system, making you more prone to infections, poor health and disease. It can also impact you directly or indirectly. When you're in a stressful state rather than a relaxed one, you have more stress hormones circulating in your system.

Identifying Stress

By completing your life inventory, you can identify the stresses in your life, real or perceived, mental or physical. Throughout this programme, you will recreate the balance between the sympathetic and parasympathetic nervous systems.

And here is the science of mindfulness. As I've stated, your breath is a key component of this practice. Deep breathing can stimulate the vagus nerve. This switches off your stress response and the effects of adrenaline on the body, lowering your heart rate and blood pressure and producing a calming effect. Activities such as yoga and tai chi work in a similar way. It has been shown that lower levels of the stress hormone cortisol are among the many benefits of mindfulness. Like adrenaline, cortisol is released when the fight-or-flight system is activated. It switches off non-essential body functions such as the immune response and digestion so that the body is more focused on preparing for an event.

Through the act of maintaining awareness and being present, you undergo a mental reprogramming. Mindfulness practice can therefore lead to improvements in various aspects of your life, including work, relationships and the management of stress and anxiety, which helps overall wellbeing. However, what most people do not realize is that life will continue to be full of ups and downs: no wellbeing programme can promise that you won't face any further difficulties, or that everything will be wonderful all the time. What I say with this programme is that, yes, life will throw things your way, and these things will often be beyond your control; but how you *react* to these events is within your control.

Doctor's Prescription:
Life's a Beach

The good news is that everybody has a parasympathetic nervous system – so here is a hack that you can use to promote wellbeing by indulging in activities and thoughts that will activate it. Remember, the parasympathetic nervous system cannot distinguish between what's real and what's not; so you can activate the relaxation mode through thought alone.

○ Close your eyes and bring focus to your breath.

○ You are at the beach. Feel the soft sand under your feet and the warm sun on your hands and face. You can hear the gentle ebb and flow of the water at the shoreline while you breath in the salty beach air.

○ Your breath is also in a calm state of ebb and flow, in and out.

○ You feel a serenity and calmness here. No thing or person demands your attention.

○ Stay here as long as you need, while your worries drift away with the ocean waves.

You don't need to go and buy an expensive holiday to feel relaxed. If you use all your senses in visualization and truly imagine being at the beach, your body will think you are there!

Neuroplasticity and Visualization

This is a wonderful feature of the brain that allows it to adapt in response to new information and experiences. In this process, new neural pathways are created. This means that our thoughts and emotions can significantly alter our brains, further highlighting the relationship between the mind and the body in overall wellbeing. The phenomenon of neuroplasticity allows you to hack your nervous system: by gaining control of your thoughts and what you feed into the brain, you can use the brain's plasticity to your advantage. Think of neuroplasticity as the rewiring of the brain in a similar way to the rewiring of an electrical circuit, or setting an alternative route on Google Maps to get to a destination.

Explaining Neuroplasticity

Neuroplasticity is our neurological response to challenges and rewards; it is involved in our ability to learn from the past and adjust to the future accordingly. In patients with depression, there is thought to be a disruption in the plasticity process. Grey matter can be boosted by exercises such as music therapy or learning a new language, which strengthen neural pathways. During rehabilitation, such as in stroke patients, the brain is encouraged to form new connections to improve motor function. The formation of new brain connections does not just happen at birth but continues throughout life. So the idea that you're too old to learn something new is scientifically incorrect!

Conversely, some neural pathways will be abolished if the brain no longer uses them. This 'pruning' explains why you might learn a language or a maths concept such as Pythagoras Theorem at school but can no longer recall them in your adult life – because you haven't revisited the information for many years, the brain has eliminated it.

The fundamental pillar of neuroplasticity is repetition. This strengthens the pathways that we wish to create. The theory is that old negative habits will be eradicated with the formation of new pathways, and triggers that previously set you off on a downward spiral will not have the same effect. There are additional steps you can take to boost this process. Ensuring you get enough sleep is vital. Sleep allows the brain to improve neuronal growth, which helps with the transmission of information. Exercise also promotes new neuronal formation.

Your nervous system loves to associate and remember the past. So, any triggers become imprinted in our DNA as a protective mechanism. For example, if a certain food causes you to have severe diarrhoea and vomiting, you will probably avoid it. Even though eating that food may not make you unwell in the future, your internal system has learned to associate it with an unpleasant reaction. Emerging research has shown that through meditation and mindfulness, these associations can be overcome.

In the lemon exercise mentioned earlier in the book (see page 54), I have already demonstrated how conjuring mental images can have a physical effect on your body, because the body cannot distinguish between what is real and imaginary. In fact, 90 per cent of the information processed by the brain is from visual stimuli, and the brain processes pictures 60,000 times faster than text. A patient is more likely to remember what they see during a consultation than what they hear – which is why in most consultations I like to give patients leaflets to use as a reference, rather than asking them to just remember what we spoke about. This is also supported by the Instagram generation, where it is reported that 82 per cent of people prefer to watch a video rather than read a social-media post.

Images provide a much easier way to digest information, especially complex data. If I tell a patient about their osteoarthritis, describing in detail the wear and tear of the bones and lack of synovial fluid, this will not be as effective as drawing a picture of their joint and the effect of the condition on the body in relation to their symptoms. Visual data enables a clearer and quicker understanding of the problem.

Explaining Visualization

Visualization is an integral part of mindfulness work. It can support personal goals by encouraging the participant to have a clear image in their mind of what they wish to achieve.

Neuroplasticity and visualization go hand in hand. It's well known that top-performing world-class athletes use visualization techniques in their training. World heavyweight boxing legend Muhammad Ali referred to visualization as 'future history'. Before each fight, he would picture in his head many times over how the match would go; and most of his bouts indeed went the way he'd mentally rehearsed.

Gold-medallist skier Lindsey Vonn attributes her success to visualization. However, not only does she visualize each ski run beforehand, including the twists and turns; she also uses her whole body to immerse herself in the visual image – physically moving back and forth as if she were on skis and incorporating breathing patterns to strengthen her visualization technique.

This sort of mental training is now widely used in rehabilitation medicine. In their 2004 study looking at the effects of mental training on strength, Vinoth K. Ranganathan and colleagues showed that internal imagery produces physiological responses in the body such as elevated breathing, heart rate and blood pressure; and that during visualization cortical centres in the brain are activated, affecting motor control, attention, planning and memory. This means that the body is better equipped to undertake an activity. As this study demonstrated, just visualizing doing the exercises resulted in increased muscle strength.

Like neuroplasticity, the more a mental image is repeated, the stronger its imprint in your brain. Thinking about a stressful event will activate your sympathetic nervous system in the same way as if you were physically experiencing that stressful event. The key to visualization practice is imagining that you've already fulfilled whatever goal you wish to achieve. So, rather than thinking about it happening in the future, you're living the goal in the present moment. With visualization, you are in control instead of living your life reacting to your environment.

How to Visualize

1. **Set a goal.** Be specific – for example, 'I want my productivity to increase by 15 per cent'; 'I want to get an A-star in maths'; 'I want to run 200 metres'.

2. **Create affirmations to boost your practice.** These are specific statements that relate to your goals, using language that aligns with the desired outcome. So, your affirmations wouldn't say that you 'hope' for something, because that would mean you'd always be stuck in the 'hope' phase. Instead, affirmations should reflect the idea that you've already achieved your goal so that your body and mind align to that 'reality'. For example, if your goal is 'I want my productivity to increase by 15 per cent', your affirmation might be, 'My productivity has increased by 15 per cent.' Likewise, 'I want to lose 5 kilos' becomes 'I am my desired weight'.

3. **Use mental pictures.** You might also use a vision board (whether physical or digital) that supports your goals – for example, featuring pictures of a country you wish to visit, a company you wish to work for, or an ideal body shape.

4. **Involve the five senses.** Use your sight, smell, touch, taste and hearing. This will trick your brain even further into believing that what you are visualizing is real. So, if you're thinking about a holiday, feel the warm sun on your arms, the touch of the sand on your feet, the sound of the seagulls, the taste of the salty

sea water and the beautiful image of a sunset reflected in the ocean. The more detail you add, the better. Needless to say, you should be closing your eyes while doing a visualization.

5. **Consider the mind–body and heart relationship.** We want to make this experience as real as possible, so we need to add emotion to the experience. So if for example you are imagining speaking in front of a large audience, incorporate feelings of success and confidence while you're mentally rehearsing.

If you don't know what it is that you want in life, then I suggest revisiting the life-inventory task earlier in the programme (see page 30). Alternatively, look at various aspects of your life and think about where you would like to make improvements, and then rank them according to how important they are to you. This might relate to your career, your health, finances, the place where you live, relationships and family, hobbies or the local community. Try to find a time in the day when you're not feeling overwhelmed and have no pressing engagements. You'll want to take time to do this without feeling rushed. The most effective times will be just as you wake up, before you enter the doing mode, or just before going to sleep, knowing that everything has been done for the day and you are closer to a relaxed state.

Getting to your desired goal may involve taking a series of appropriate steps. This could mean finding out more information – so taking a course, hiring someone with expertise, or just conducting your own general research. You may wish to outline the steps and visualize each one. There are many free guided visualizations online that would supplement this practice. You might look for ones specifically aligned with your goal – for example, visualizations for weightloss.

Watch out for your self-critic. If you imagine you've won £10,000 and your monkey chatter starts to ridicule you, remember: there are no limits to your imagination, but when you start to doubt yourself, the brain will not accept the suggestions as readily. To overcome this doubt, just be aware of the thoughts without getting caught up in them. Let them just float away, without judging yourself as a failure, and then carry on with the visualization.

Lecturer Tim Blankert and Professor Melvyn Hamstra developed a specific type of imagery that is now considered to be the most effective form of visualization. It's called PETTLEP, which means:

◇ Physical
◇ Environmental
◇ Task
◇ Timing
◇ Learning
◇ Emotional
◇ Perspective

All these aspects should be part of the visualization process. Adopting the PETTLEP method encourages the brain to view it as more realistic. This is a bit like the difference between playing a video game with poor graphics and playing one with realistic effects – you're likely to enjoy the realistic one more.

Doctor's Prescription:
Release of Muscle Tension and Tightness

Stress can often manifest as physical tension. In fact, it's like a reflex action where the body protects itself: if the stress is acute, the muscle goes back to its resting state. However, this does not occur in chronic stress and consequently the area affected can extend. For example, if you have chronic headaches then your neck and upper back may also become affected.

An effective exercise to release muscle stress and promote muscle relaxation is to tense and then release different muscles.

○ Start at the top and take a deep breath in. Then begin to tense your face by screwing it up tightly, including your eyes, for thirty seconds; then release with a big sigh.

○ Work your way down to your shoulders: hunch them towards you and then release.

○ Next, flex your arms tightly and release.

○ Finish with the legs and toes.

○ Finally, just sit for a few moments, feeling totally relaxed and with your breath.

The Flow State

You may have heard this being referred to as 'being in the zone'. It describes a state where a person is fully engaged and immersed in the activity they're doing, with their senses heightened. In the flow state, it's as if you've lost yourself in the task to such a degree that you have no awareness of time or the world around you. You may have experienced this when spending time with friends, absorbed in a good book or watching a sports game, painting, playing a musical instrument, or even scrolling through social media.

The term originated from psychologist Mihály Csíkszentmihály, who described it as the secret to happiness. So, how does the flow state relate to wellbeing and mindfulness? They have a very close relationship in terms of learning: in both mindfulness and the flow state you are fully present and both lead to feelings of enjoyment or fulfilment. Think of mindfulness as a pathway to achieving a flow state, where the internal monkey chatter, negative thoughts, feelings of boredom, pain, tiredness and hunger dissipate.

Amy Isham and Professor Tim Jackson at the Centre for Understanding Sustainable Prosperity, University of Surrey, say: 'flow experiences are linked to higher levels of personal wellbeing and appear to be more likely to occur during activities that are less environmentally costly.' The benefit of achieving a flow state is that the heightened focus and concentration will increase the efficiency of whatever task you're doing.

Letting Go of Doing

This improves the learning process. Most of the time, you will be focused on living your life in the doing mode. This is task-orientated with deadlines. So rather than going for a walk in the evening just to improve your health, you'll go only to achieve the number of steps or exercise hours you've set yourself. Today we have become quite obsessed with targets even outside the work environment. However, while this mindset certainly allows you to achieve your goals, it is perpetuating that sympathetic stressful pathway.

Think of the flow-state concept as an extra boost to your wellbeing programme. It can help you develop the skills to regulate your emotions and provide you with motivation to do things that make you feel inwardly and outwardly happy. In that zone, you'll immediately feel a sense of positivity. It will also help you overcome the feelings of self-doubt and worthlessness that often hold you back from undertaking activities. There is varied research into how these effects come about. One school of thought suggests that during the flow state there is an increase of dopamine, which is involved in pleasure and reward.

The flow state and mindfulness are like two pieces of a jigsaw – and similar principles apply. Entering a flow state requires a similar process to beginning a formal meditation practice – therefore first ensure that you eliminate distractions so you can give the task your full attention. Rather than multitasking, be specific about what it is that you plan to do; this could involve setting a clear goal that is both attainable and doable. It's also important to ensure the activity is something that you enjoy. The task can be something simple, such as taking a bath or doing physical exercise.

Doctor's Prescription:
The Flow State

To incorporate mindfulness into achieving a flow state for an activity:

- Bring to mind the specific goal or activity you are about to undertake.

- Start to pay attention to your breath to build your focus and free yourself from any self-doubt.

- Now bring your full attention and awareness to the task.

- Check in with yourself while undertaking the task

to see if any negative thoughts have crept in or if your attention has wandered. If it has, bring yourself back to the present moment without criticism. Giving a commentary may help you. For example, 'I am now running; I am using my muscles; I can sense the ground ...'

When you have finished the task, reflect on your experience and how you're feeling. There may be something you'd like to change next time to make it more productive. This could be something simple, like checking the weather forecast before digging the garden.

Dealing with Setbacks in Your Journey

Your wellbeing journey is no different to any other journey, in that you will have moments of progress as well as challenging times. Mindfulness involves freeing yourself from labels such as 'perfection'. We keep a realistic outlook, and our focus should be on how to respond to such challenges.

When faced with setbacks, you could adopt them and tell yourself, 'This always happens to me,' or, 'I knew this was going to happen,' feeding into thoughts of low self-esteem and low self-worth. However, if we instead view challenges as opportunities for learning and growth then they can in fact provide a catalyst for wellbeing. Such moments allow us to reflect and focus on what went well and what didn't go so well, keeping in mind that any journey requires flexibility. The number or nature of setbacks is not related to your potential for growth. This mental reframing is essential to your ability to cope.

Fostering a Growth Mindset

Adopting a growth mindset and compassion may involve adjusting or delaying your goals and expectation. For example, rather than trying to complete a 10,000-word project in one go, you may want to make it more manageable and commit to writing 5,000 words each week. If you're having difficulty in writing, you may set yourself a goal to speak to an expert in the field. Rather than trying to lose 1 kilo in two weeks, you may need to factor in upcoming social occasions or life events and focus not on weightloss as a number but rather on small wins such as portion control or having fewer sugary snacks.

Resilience plays an important role in evaluating setbacks in your journey. Resilience, empathy, and a positive mindset are all skills that will naturally become stronger through a mindfulness programme. Resilience in this situation will allow you to have the right mental and physical skills to cope with and, more importantly, to recover from challenges.

When training medical students to become doctors, we tell them that mistakes can happen – whether it's misplacing a report or losing a sample of blood. The way to deal with these mistakes is to first be honest and secondly take ownership. It is also essential to be solution-focused rather than dwelling on the problem. This ensures that lessons are learned so that the mistake does not happen again while also taking the necessary steps to rectify it. This process of reflection is crucial and adds to your progress rather than hindering it. Through following a similar exercise in your own journey, you will learn more about yourself and identify blocks to your progress. There will be days that your determination will waver; allow yourself to have those moments, but don't dwell on them too long. Using the principles of mindfulness, the first step is to acknowledge how you're feeling and adjust accordingly to continue your wellbeing journey with renewed optimism.

Ten Steps for Dealing with Setbacks

1. **Recognize the difficulty that you're in.** This involves acknowledging your feelings, which may range from upset to angry to frustrated or disappointed.
2. **Cultivate compassion.** Rather than berating yourself, take comfort in the knowledge that every person experiences setbacks and that they're not a sign of failure.
3. **Reframe.** This is a space for learning and moving forward.
4. **Reflect.** Identify any factors that led to the difficulty.
5. **Recover.** Having identified obstacles, evaluate how you might overcome these or do things differently next time.
6. **Pause.** You may need a break from this aspect of your life; you can return with renewed energy another day to tackle it again.
7. **Strengthen your coping mechanisms.** This includes ensuring that you have adequate sleep, a healthy diet and regular exercise.
8. **Communicate.** Discuss how you're feeling with others. You may find that certain colleagues or friends are more supportive than others. Notice this. Build

your relationships with them, so that you can help them in their times of need too.

9. **Journalling.** There may be lingering thoughts of self-doubt and negativity. If you don't feel comfortable discussing these with others, your journal is a safe space to put your thoughts on paper.

10. **Gratitude.** Give thanks for every learning opportunity and to those in your circle who have helped you overcome your challenges.

Doctor's Prescription:
Learning Versus Performance

Remind yourself that every challenge is transitory. The phrase 'This too shall pass' is probably one of the most significant to our wellbeing journey.

To cultivate a growth mindset, adopt goals that are learning-focused rather than performance-focused. This involves freeing yourself from creating list upon list of endless targets and beating yourself up if you don't achieve them.

This will shift the emphasis to the process of learning and self-improvement, which will then provide the necessary skills to tackle anything that comes your way. You'll also avoid labels such as 'failure', which promote negativity.

For example, say you have an exam and your goal is to achieve a particular grade. Reframe the goal as developing effective study techniques so that you're equipped for any exam.

Keeping Your Camp Upright

You have reached the end of this guide, the purpose of which was to work with your mind so that you can undo the mental programming that's held you back for so long, as well as acknowledging your heart so that your journey is truly nourishing and holistic. Like any troubleshooting guide, you'll need to refer back to this in turbulent times. Repetition is key, so this is not a book you just read once. This programme requires work.

This book places much emphasis on the prevention of difficulties. However, it will be just as useful when challenges arise. Consistency is key and so is awareness – noticing the small gains that accumulate into significant changes in your life. This is a marathon and not a sprint: this programme isn't designed to be a quick-fix guide; instead, it's something you can refer back to for many years to come.

Just as a camp provides shelter from unpredictable weather and the unknowns of the wilderness, this guide aims to foster a sense of stability and resilience so that you can navigate the challenges ahead while still experiencing joy and happiness. The camp symbolizes a space in which you can safely reflect and build necessary tools within yourself to achieve your goals.

Notice when the camp needs strengthening. If a frame comes loose, you have the tools and equipment to fix it and regain control. The camp cannot simply be erected and stay like that by magic throughout the storm; it needs your awareness and effort. But this is very achievable – with practice, fixing the camp will become second nature.

The hardest part is setting up a camp from scratch. Once erected, however, your camp will provide you with strength, mirroring the conscious effort you have made by staying with this guide. Now that you are here, remind yourself that the camp will provide comfort whenever you need it. In time, you can venture further and further away from it with confidence, knowing you can return to it if the weather pattern becomes gloomy again.

I love giving my patients lists and action plans at the end of a consultation. I feel it gives them direction and makes things feel much more manageable; in this digital age, things can too often feel overwhelming.

Five Tips to Keep Your Camp Upright

1. **Return to the present moment.** A mind that is occupied with past regrets or future anxiety is a mind that can never foster wellbeing.
2. **Incorporate heart-based living.** While much is

known about the mind–body connection, a life based on compassion and love allows a deeper connection with yourself and others in your life, leading to fulfilment.

3. **Be here for lifelong learning.** Ditch the idea that there is a one-stop shop that will fix all your problems. Welcome instead the rest of your life, where you will be constantly learning. Keep engaged with this process through informal and formal mindfulness practices, recognizing that there is no ceiling to your potential and growth.

4. **Listen.** There is one person who can give you a unique perspective and insight into your wellbeing journey and that is you. Pay attention to your thoughts that try to hinder your progress and forget the gains, of which there will be many. Listen to your physical body too; acknowledge its limits and supplement your journey with adequate sleep, diet and exercise.

5. **It's about you.** The central theme of this book is that you take a proactive step into your happiness, having the confidence to take charge of your journey as well as the destination. Through the work here, you will get to know yourself, your triggers and your motivations in a way that no one else can. Know that you can instigate a change in your life and overcome challenges. To do this requires prioritizing your self-care and patience.

Doctor's Prescription:
Diaphragmatic Breathing

There are times when you need an instant relief from stress. The most practical way is to use the tools you have already. Diaphragmatic breathing is a simple yet effective method for relaxation.

○ Sit with your feet flat on the floor in a quiet place.

○ Put one hand on your upper chest and the other on the top of your abdomen (above the belly button).

○ Take a deep breath in through your nose and allow your abdomen to push your hand away.

○ Breathe out through your mouth and allow your abdomen to shrink back in towards you.

○ Continue this for a minimum of five minutes.

The diaphragm muscle is located at the base of the lungs and is doing the work here by controlling the nervous system and therefore promoting relaxation. The chest is not involved, so it stays still throughout.

Meditations

Meditations for the final week are to ensure that your camp is strong and can withstand life's challenges. Throughout this programme, the focus of these meditations can remind you that you can shape your healing journey – you just need to show up.

The Light

Regardless of whether you're new to meditation or an experienced meditator, sometimes you just need to start right back at the beginning. This is the perfect meditation to begin your meditation journey. It's also a great illuminative exercise with which to open your day, or to lighten your load and help you relax into a state ready for a peaceful night's sleep.

1. Prepare yourself and your surroundings and free yourself from the concept of time. Give yourself

permission to devote this moment to nothing but yourself.

2. This is the most compassionate and effective way to settle your nervous system. Notice where you feel the breath the most, where it captures your attention the most. This may be around your nose, or your mouth, in the rise and fall of the chest wall or in your abdomen.

3. Your breath does not need your manipulation; it is a delicate, intricate system that knows exactly what to do, without any interference from your self-critic.

4. As you stay with the breath, your mind will continue to try to control the narrative. It is uncomfortable when you do not give it attention. It will try to distract you with thoughts. Thoughts of the past, thoughts of the future ... Planning. Reminiscing. Analysing.

5. But there is no need to judge yourself harshly, because this is the way of the mind. In fact, offer the mind compassion and kindness for doing what it knows best, with the intention of being in a survival mode. Awareness that your mind has wandered is enough at this moment. Gently, and without criticism of yourself, bring your awareness back to the breath.

6. Pay attention to the character of the breath. Is it shallow or deep? Have you noticed that your breath has naturally slowed down during this practice, as the sympathetic nervous system begins to shut down and you enter a biochemical relaxation state? With the slowing down of the respiration rate, your heart rate will follow its friend and slow down too, knowing that your bodily systems are all connected.

7. You are now in a deeply nourishing state. You are

allowing your body to rest and recover. Intentionally rejuvenate yourself with a light that extends from your crown to the very tips of your toes. This is self-compassion at its most effective.

8. In this moment of stillness, you are providing your physical body and mental health with the healing they deserve. A chance to be at peace, for your mind to settle. Without rushing to be anywhere, not thinking about doing something; just basking in the awareness of the body and the breath.

9. In this moment, you will feel full – full of life, full of tranquillity, replacing the emptiness you felt before. There is an ease. There is spaciousness. There is an openness.

10. You may feel that some areas are still closed, feeling tight, or that the mind wants you to focus on areas of discomfort – maybe your lower back, some remaining tension in the jaw, or stiffness in the neck perhaps. Notice this. It's already on your mind. Breathe into those areas. Let them feel relaxation. Stay in these areas for as long as you need to. Breathing in, breathing out. Nourishing those body parts with revitalizing oxygen.

11. When you are ready to draw this meditative practice to a close, take one more deep breath in and a longer exhalation out. Open your eyes if you need to; adjust your posture as your body requires.

The Circulatory System

Your circulatory system is made up of blood vessels that carry blood towards the heart and then deliver vital nutrients, hormones and oxygen to the whole body. It is in perfect balance, keeping the travel in one direction and supporting your very being.

1. Close your eyes and as you sit here focus your attention on the heart. Show appreciation for how tirelessly it works. Feel the steady rhythm as it beats, pumping blood throughout your body.
2. The heart is the centre of your being, carrying life-force energy to every single cell. Place your hands over your heart to increase your connection with it.
3. Visualize the heart contracting and then relaxing in an effortless flow, working in harmony with the breath. Everything is in perfect equilibrium.
4. Draw energy from this powerful muscle and let it radiate throughout your being.
5. Now you have shown appreciation for the physical role it plays, show gratitude for its spiritual role as it allows you to feel love and compassion. Feel this energy now spreading from the heart to your crown, then down to your feet.
6. In this moment, you can let go of all the demands and expectations and become your true self as you focus on the heart, which brings all your internal systems together.
7. There are about 40,000 neurons in the heart that can feel, learn and sense. This is a place of openness and security, where fears can be left behind.

8. Often the mind overrides the inputs from the heart, but the heart is a place of great wisdom. Use its lessons to appreciate and care for others and express kindness to those around you.

9. Through gratitude and acknowledgement of the heart, you now bring it into balance with your mind – providing you with equanimity and stability in your life.

The Cloak

There is a cloak in your life that shelters you from harm, keeping you safe and secure from the many challenges that you face. If you are feeling particularly vulnerable or anxious, this meditation will help alleviate those feelings.

1. Close your eyes. Visualize yourself standing in a street. Notice the cars, houses, the streetlamp, and the wind causing a faint rustling of the leaves.

2. You feel a slight chill standing here. This represents your mind, which has some specific worries and concerns. Bring them to the forefront.

3. Observe them as a bystander on the road, rather than getting enveloped in those thoughts and emotions.

4. A person approaches. As they get closer, you notice it is someone familiar – someone who you love and who provides comfort.

5. You feel a sense of relief. They have in their hand a huge draping cloak. They place this on your shoulders, and you feel its velvety texture, immediately providing you with warmth.

6. For extra security, the cloak is fastened loosely but firmly around your neck. Now you feel the added wisdom and knowledge it provides.
7. What you were troubled by is no longer part of you. You notice the distance between you and the concern.
8. With this protective energy around your being, you feel a deep connection to your higher self. Take some deep breaths and recall all the wealthy and powerful figures in history wearing cloaks, from royalty to leaders of the most powerful army. This state of being fulfils you throughout.
9. With a sense of freedom, you turn to head home, walking with a spring in your step – with renewed vitality and energy, knowing you can face any difficulties ahead with ease.

The Wind That Scatters

Nature sounds are known to promote a feeling of relaxation. Thinking of the wind creates a powerful image of your troubles being released high up into the air, far away, never to come back.

1. Visualize the energy of wind, gently flowing, entering your being and being part of your breath.
2. Breathe in and breathe out with the calm nature of the wind. The wind nourishes every bit of you as it is carried by the breath to each part of the body.
3. The breath of the wind reaches the crown of your head. Stay present here. You notice your thoughts and emotions are a chaotic whirlwind.

4. As you continue to breathe, the wind begins to scatter those thoughts that are causing you concern.
5. As a clearing forms in your mind, you feel a sense of calmness and serenity.
6. The wind carries away the worries, doubts and negative thoughts that have been consuming you. The landscape has changed. You feel open and light.
7. Take some final deep breaths with the power of the healing wind. Let those worries dissipate into the surrounding air, carried far away from you.

Morning Mindfulness

Set your morning with a calm and clear mindset. You are in control of how your day unfolds. Try to do this exercise instead of reaching for your phone, which will activate the sympathetic nervous system.

1. Close your eyes and start to take some deep and slow breaths. Notice those first breaths that you take in the morning, filling your lungs and every part of your body.
2. With each breath, continue to relax deeper and deeper, softening any areas of tension or tightness you feel from the night before.
3. Welcome this new day as it provides new opportunities for growth. Through the breath, you have created space for learning and love.
4. Bring to mind any activities you need to do during the day ahead.
5. Visualize each task going smoothly and positively, without challenges. Notice how you feel about having

accomplished all that you set out to do.

6. With the intuition of the heart and the wisdom of your mind, let your whole being involve itself in the success that will follow this day.

7. Trust in yourself that there will be many moments today for which you will be grateful.

8. With vitality and renewed energy, slowly begin to open your eyes fully, ready for the day ahead.

Informal Mindfulness Practice

Reflect on This Week

Recall a practice or skill that you did this week. Then ask yourself the following questions and write down the answers:

- ◇ What went well?
- ◇ How did it make you feel?
- ◇ Did you notice any changes in your life, however small?
- ◇ What could you have improved on?

Mindful Showering

Suggested time: ten minutes daily.

These informal mindfulness practices are designed to incorporate everyday tasks into your wellbeing process by bringing awareness and staying in the present moment, rather than being caught up in the past or future.

1. Feel the water on your skin. Notice the temperature and the texture.
2. See the water as it falls from the shower head just like raindrops.
3. Smell the scent of the soap, and notice the texture of the soft lather as it forms a foam on your skin.
4. Hear the water drifting away along with the day's tension and troubles.
5. You now feel truly revitalized and refreshed.

END OF WEEK FIVE

Week Five, the final week. But also the beginning. This is the start of a new journey with a renewed outlook and inner tools to promote your wellbeing and independence.

Afterword

After twenty years of practising medicine, I understand the physical and emotional challenges that individuals face. Yet the solutions aren't always so clear to patients, and much work is needed in the areas of disease prevention and health promotion.

When I began to write this book, I was torn between talking to you as though you're one of the hundreds of patients I've seen over the years or as your friend, guide, or mentor. In the end, I wrote this book using a combination of all those perspectives.

My final words for you all are to remind you that your wellbeing will always be an ongoing process rather than a destination. However, as you incorporate mindfulness and self-healing into your life, that journey becomes easier. I hope this book serves as a guiding light, shining down on the camp that you have built for yourself.

Remember, the tools of mindful healing will always be with you, in your breath and in your awareness.

Stay present and hold tightly to gratitude.

I'm rooting for you.

Dr Afrosa Ahmed

Bibliography

BOOKS

Albers, S., *Eat, Drink, and be Mindful: How to End Your Struggle with Mindless Eating and Start Savoring Food with Intention and Joy* (New Harbinger, 2009)

Burch, V., *Living Well with Pain and Illness: The Mindful Way to Free Yourself from Suffering* (Sounds True, 2010)

Burch, V. and Penman, D., *Mindfulness for Health: A Practical Guide to Relieving Pain, Reducing Stress and Restoring Wellbeing* (Piatkus, 2013).

Csikszentmihalyi, M., *Flow: The Psychology of Happiness*, (Rider, 2002)

Goleman, D., Emotional Intelligence: *Why it Can Matter More Than IQ: 25th Anniversary Edition* (Bloomsbury, 2020)

Hasson, G. and Butler D., *Mental Health and Wellbeing in the Workplace: A Practical Guide for Employers and Employees: A Practical Guide for Employers and Employees* (Capstone, 2020)

Kabat-Zinn, J., *Coming To Our Senses: Healing Ourselves and the World Through Mindfulness* (Piatkus, 2005)

Kabat-Zinn, J., *Full Catastrophe Living, Revised Edition: How to Cope with Stress, Pain and Illness using Mindfulness Meditation* (Piatkus, 2013)

Kabat-Zinn, J., *Wherever You Go, There You Are: Mindfulness Meditation for Everyday Life* (Piatkus, 2004)

Maltz, M. (1960), *Psycho-Cybernetics*. New York: Simon & Schuster.

Siegel, D. J. and Payne Bryson, T., *No-Drama Discipline: the Bestselling Parenting Guide to Nurturing Your Child's Developing Mind* (Scribe UK, 2015)

Stahl, B., *A Mindfulness-Based Stress Reduction Workbook* (New Harbinger, 2019)

Williams, M. and Penman, D., *Mindfulness: A Practical Guide to Finding Peace in a Frantic World* (Piatkus, 2011)

Williams, M., Teasdale J., Segal Z. and Kabat-Zinn J., *The Mindful Way Through Depression: Freeing Yourself from Chronic Unhappiness* (Guilford Press, 2007)

JOURNAL ARTICLES

Algoe, S. (2023), 'Why It's Important to Show Gratitude at Work – and What's the Best Way to Do It', *The Wall Street Journal*.

Baikie, K.A. and Wilhelm, K. (2005), 'Emotional and physical health benefits of expressive writing', Advances in Psychiatric Treatment: The Royal College of Psychiatrists' *Journal of Continuing Professional Development*, 11(5), pp. 338–346.

Brewer, J.A. et al. (2011), 'Meditation experience is associated with differences in default mode network activity and connectivity', *Proceedings of the National Academy of Sciences* – PNAS, 108(50), pp. 20254–20259.

Butler, L. et al. (2022), 'Evidence and strategies for including emotional intelligence in pharmacy education', *American Journal of Pharmaceutical Education*, 86(10), pp. ajpe8674-1113.

Caballero, C. et al. (2019) 'Greater mindfulness is associated with better academic achievement in middle school', *Mind, Brain and Education*, 13(3), pp. 157–166.

Calcabrini, A. et al. (2004), 'Terpinen-4-ol, the main component of Melaleuca alternifolia (tea tree) oil inhibits the in vitro growth of human melanoma cells', *Journal of Investigative Dermatology*, 122, pp. 349–360.

Fioravanti, G. et al. (2023), 'Examining the impact of daily exposure to body-positive and fitspiration Instagram content on young women's mood and body image: An intensive longitudinal study', *New Media & Society*, 25(12), pp. 3266–3288.

Fox, G. R. et al. (2015), 'Neural correlates of gratitude', *Frontiers in Psychology*, 6, pp. 1491–1491.

Glass, O. et al. (2019), 'Expressive writing to improve resilience to trauma: A clinical feasibility trial', *Complementary Therapies in Clinical Practice*, 34, pp. 240–246.

Goldsby, T. L. et al. (2017), 'Effects of singing bowl sound meditation on mood, tension, and well-being: An observational study', *Journal of Evidence-Based Complementary & Alternative Medicine*, 22(3), pp. 401–406.

Goldsmith, K. and Dhar, R. (2013), 'Negativity bias and task motivation: Testing the effectiveness of positively versus negatively framed incentives', *Journal of Experimental Psychology. Applied*, 19(4), pp. 358–366.

Gordon, A.M. et al. (2012), 'To Have and to Hold: Gratitude Promotes Relationship Maintenance in Intimate Bonds', *Journal of Personality and Social Psychology*, 103(2), pp. 257–274.

Harvard Medical School (2011), 'Mindfulness meditation practice changes the brain', *Harvard Women's Health Watch*, 18(8), pp. 6–.

Hölzel, B. K. et al. (2011) 'Mindfulness practice leads to increases in regional brain gray matter density', *Psychiatry Research*, 191(1), pp. 36–43.

Hsu, H.-P. (2021), 'The Psychological Meaning of Self-Forgiveness in a Collectivist Context and the Measure Development', *Psychology Research and Behavior Management*, 14, pp. 2059–2069.

Kakoschke, N. et al. (2021), 'The importance of formal versus informal mindfulness practice for enhancing psychological wellbeing and study engagement in a medical student cohort with a 5-week mindfulness-based lifestyle program', PLOS ONE, 16(10), pp. e0258999–e0258999.

Kalan, A.K., Kulik, L., Arandjelovic, M. et al. (2020), 'Environmental variability supports chimpanzee behavioural diversity', *Nature Communications*, 11, 4451.

Kubzansky, L. D. et al. (2018), 'Positive psychological well-being and cardiovascular disease: JACC health-promotion series', *Journal of the American College of Cardiology*, 72(12), pp. 1382–1396.

Levine, N. et al. (2001), 'Psychological health, well-being, and the mind-heart-body connection: A scientific statement from the American Heart Association', *Circulation*, 143(10), pp. e763–e783.

Malinowski, P. and Lim, H. J. (2015), 'Mindfulness at Work: Positive Affect, Hope, and Optimism Mediate the Relationship Between Dispositional Mindfulness, Work Engagement, and Well-Being', *Mindfulness*, 6(6), pp. 1250–1262.

Mauger, P. A., Perry, J. E., Freeman, T., Grove, D. C., et al. (1992), 'The measurement of forgiveness: Preliminary research', *Journal of Psychology and Christianity*, 11(2), 170–180.

McCullough, M. E. et al. (1998), 'Interpersonal Forgiving in Close Relationships: II. Theoretical Elaboration and Measurement', *Journal of Personality and Social Psychology*, 75(6), pp. 1586–1603.

Naghdi, L. et al. (2015), 'The effect of low-frequency sound stimulation on patients with fibromyalgia: A clinical study', *Pain Research & Management*, 20(1), pp. E21–E27.

Ranganathan, V. K. et al. (2004), 'From mental power to muscle power—gaining strength by using the mind', *Neuropsychologia*, 42(7), pp. 944–956.

Smit, B. and Stavrulaki, E. (2021), 'The Efficacy of a Mindfulness-Based Intervention for College Students Under Extremely Stressful Conditions', *Mindfulness*, 12(12), pp. 3086–3100.

Stone S. and Bernstein M. (2007), 'Prospective error recording in surgery: an analysis of 1108 elective neurosurgical cases', *Neurosurgery*, 60(6):1075-80.

Waters, L. and Stokes, H. (2015), 'Positive education for school leaders: exploring the effects of emotion-gratitude and action-gratitude', *The Australian Educational and Developmental Psychologist*, 32(1), pp. 1–22.

Wegner, D. M. et al. (1987), 'Paradoxical Effects of Thought Suppression', *Journal of Personality and Social Psychology*, 53(1), pp. 5–13.

Wendt, S. et al. (2015), 'Practicing transcendental meditation in high schools: Relationship to well-being and academic achievement among students', *Contemporary School Psychology*, 19(4), pp. 312–319.

Wohl, M. J. A., Pychyl, T. A. and Bennett, S. H. (2010), 'I forgive myself, now I can study: How self-forgiveness for procrastinating can reduce future procrastination', *Personality and Individual Differences*, 48(7), pp. 803–808.

Wong, Y. J. et al. (2018), 'Does gratitude writing improve the mental health of psychotherapy clients? Evidence from a randomized controlled trial', *Psychotherapy Research*, 28(2), pp. 192–202.

Yu, L. and Zellmer-Bruhn, M. (2018), 'Introducing team mindfulness and considering its safeguard role against conflict transformation and social undermining', *Academy of Management Journal*, 61(1), pp. 324–347.

Yusuf, S. et al.; INTERHEART Study Investigators (2004), 'Effect of potentially modifiable risk factors associated with myocardial infarction in 52 countries (the INTERHEART study): Case-control study', *Lancet*, 364(9438), pp. 937–52.

Zahn, R. et al. (2009), 'The neural basis of human social values: Evidence from functional MRI', *Cerebral Cortex*, 19(2), pp. 276–283.

USEFUL WEBSITES

breathworks-mindfulness.org.uk

oxfordmindfulness.org

bangor.ac.uk/centre-for-mindfulness

mindfulnessinschools.org/mindfulness-in-education/

jonkabat-zinn.com

mbsrtraining.com

franticworld.com

home.mindfulness-network.org

mindfulnessnow.org.uk